A Thousand Worries

SUNY series in Black Women's Wellness
—————
Stephanie Y. Evans, editor

A Thousand Worries

Black Women Mothering Autistic Sons

JEANNINE E. DINGUS-EASON

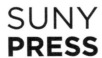

Published by State University of New York Press, Albany

© 2024 State University of New York

All rights reserved

Printed in the United States of America

No part of this book may be used or reproduced in any manner whatsoever without written permission. No part of this book may be stored in a retrieval system or transmitted in any form or by any means including electronic, electrostatic, magnetic tape, mechanical, photocopying, recording, or otherwise without the prior permission in writing of the publisher.

For information, contact State University of New York Press, Albany, NY
www.sunypress.edu

Library of Congress Cataloging-in-Publication Data

Name: Dingus-Eason, Jeannine E., author.
Title: A thousand worries : Black women mothering autistic sons / Jeannine E. Dingus-Eason.
Description: Albany : State University of New York Press, [2024]. | Series: SUNY series in Black women's wellness | Includes bibliographical references and index.
Identifiers: LCCN 2023019218 | ISBN 9781438496122 (hardcover : alk. paper) | ISBN 9781438496146 (ebook) | ISBN 9781438496139 (pbk. : alk. paper)
Subjects: LCSH: Autistic children. | Mothers of autistic children. | African American mothers.
Classification: LCC HQ773.8 .D56 2024 | DDC 305.9/084083—dc23/eng/20231030
LC record available at https://lccn.loc.gov/2023019218

10 9 8 7 6 5 4 3 2 1

*To Caleb,
Gamommy,
Gram
&
Uncle Jerry*

But by the grace of God I am what I am, and his grace to me was not without effect. No, I worked harder than all of them—yet not I, but the grace of God that was with me.

—1 Corinthians 15:10

Contents

Acknowledgments		xi
Prelude: "I Am Caleb's Mom"		xv
Introduction		1
Chapter 1	Study Overview	9
Chapter 2	The Making of Black Autism Mothers	27
Chapter 3	"Black Mommas Need Action Items"	43
Chapter 4	Black Mothers at the Intersection of Race, Class, Gender, and Autism	69
Chapter 5	Education at the Intersection of Race, Class, Gender, and Autism	93
Chapter 6	Black Is the New Autism: BAMs and Autism Representation	117
Chapter 7	BAMs and the Future	147
Conclusion		167
Afterword		189
References		195
Index		211

Acknowledgments

I am abundantly blessed to have so many caring, thoughtful individuals surrounding me. You helped breathe life into this book, bolstered me, and encouraged my vision. A special thank-you is in order to my family, beginning with my dear Caleb. You are such an amazing, smart, sweet, caring young man. You inspire me to be better and move me to action. My husband, Majied, deserves a special thank-you for just being you. My writing shifts wrap up at 5:00 a.m., but you always made a point of inquiring about my progress. You take exceptionally good care of Caleb, and I and we love you dearly in return. My mother Sarah is the only one who read early drafts of chapters. You are my inspiration with your patience, kind heart, and deep abiding faith. Cousin Wanda Heath helped us along this journey. Robert Sr., your calming voice and quiet support made a difference. My siblings Karen, Renee, and Robert supported us on our journey. For this, I am eternally grateful. A thousand shouts of gratitude are not enough to thank my family: the Frasiers, Easons, Coopers, Bolers, Lewises, Dilberts (Stephanie and Terri), and the Thompsons. The Trinity Emmanuel church family has always been a source of love and support. Many thanks to the Finch family and the Millers for your abiding love for Caleb.

Many thanks to my coworkers at St. John Fisher University. Drs. Guillermo Montes, Marie Cianca, Shannon Cleverley-Thompson, Sue Schultz, and Katrina Arndt deserve special thanks for their kind words over the years. Dr. Montes laid the foundation for this work, as we shared many conversations regarding the topic of Black mothers and autism. You validated my ideas during those times of limited confidence. Special thanks to Dean Michael Wischnowski and Provost Kevin Railey for your sabbatical support. The research for this project was supported in part by

St. John Fisher University's Faculty Research Funds, which assisted with transcription and travel costs. A very special thanks to Betsy Christiansen for being one of the kindest, most efficient souls I have the privilege of knowing. I am blessed to have you in my life. I am a firm believer that people come into your life at the right time for the right reasons. My editor at State University of New York Press, Rebecca Colesworthy, is an example of that expression. She responded to my inquiries immediately and remained responsive throughout the project. Rebecca alleviated my novice writing concerns. Several reviewers shaped the book with insights, suggestions, and encouraging words. I greatly appreciate your time and detailed reviews. Your interest in the topic of Black autism mothers was genuine and that translated into your interactions with me. Thank you Stephanie Evans for your editoral support.

Special shout-outs to my scholar circle, the folks who have had my back for years, constantly pushing me to be my best. The list is extensive but includes Dr. Geneva Gay, my academic momma, who taught me that we don't do raggedy. Dr. Adrienne Dixson, my road-dog from day one. You are an extraordinarily kind, generous scholar and sister. Dr. Cory Brown for keeping the soundtrack flowing, Dr. Vanessa Dodo Seriki for your boundless creativity, and Dr. Nathalie Mizelle for your analysis. Dr. Mary Jane Curry, I thank you for being an amazing sister-ally.

My sister circle would not be complete without acknowledging my many sorors of Delta Sigma Theta Sorority, Inc. Thank you for your support in recruiting participants and your encouragement throughout the project. Your kind words made the difference. Special shout-outs to Dr. Melany Silas, Dr. Tokeya Graham, Karen Rogers, and Alerice Butler. Your assistance made all the difference! I love and adore you all! During the latter stages of composing the book, Dr. Clarissa Walker and Kimberly Conway Dumpson, who provided coaching and encouragement: you both stepped in at the right moments, pushing me to think differently about writing. Thanks to Dr. Deena Khalil who provided steady reminders that this research matters. Your words landed at the right time.

I would be remiss if I did not mention my doctoral students, who toiled along with me, simultaneously completing their dissertations. I told you *we* could do it! My Silver Vixens, Drs. Anna Rodriguez, Miriam Jurado, and Isabelle Jones: I am eternally grateful for the prayers, texts, hugs, and laughs. You three are indeed a hot mess and I aspire to be like you!! Dr. Leslie Smith also knew when to chime in with a good prayer and encouraging word. Kent Osborn deserves many thanks for a listening ear.

My Baber African Methodist Episcopal Church family, led by Rev. James C. Simmons, deserves a thank-you as well, for their unyielding support, prayers, and inquiries about the book. I love my Baber folks and there's nothing you can do about it!

Many thanks to members of Caleb's support team over the years. Miss Adrienne, Miss Elaine, Mrs. Williams, Mrs. Best, Ms. Tiffany, Mr. Brian, Mr. Sean, Mr. Gordon, Mr. Jack, Mr. Marcus, Ms. Roxanne, Ms. Jillian, Ms. Melissa, Ms. Bonnie, the House staff, Miss Martine, Dazzle, and countless others who have helped shape him into a loving young man. He has fond memories of being in your presence. Soror Henrene Brown placed us on the pathway to services and was a blessing to our family. Uncle Jerry Beckwith, whom we recently lost, was always a source of love, kindness, and consistent support.

Finally, I want to thank Black autism mothers/mommas who inspired this book, especially all participating mothers. You all are bold, creative, loving mothers!! You stepped forward without hesitation to share your experiences, your love for your sons, and your insights on mothering Black sons on the autism spectrum. I am eternally grateful to you all. Know that you are not alone. For those of you on social media: I SEE YOU. I HEAR YOU. I FEEL YOU. Stay the course and love on your babies hard!!!!

In the event that I omitted names, please charge it to my head and not my heart. Your involvement in my life and that of Caleb has shaped our autism journey. Thank you.

All praises to the Most High!

Prelude

"I Am Caleb's Mom"

"I am Caleb's mom . . ." I find myself saying these words daily. The inflection on "I" or "am," "Caleb" or "mom" differs depending on the context, the time of day, my mood, and my son's behaviors. I utter the phrase at the beginning of a sentence as a declarative statement, almost reiterating to myself the relationship between mother and child. We are eternally connected, though separated daily by the country miles between our city home and the rural group home where he resides. The words comfort me, bringing me back to my senses after some incredulous act or turn of events involving Caleb. As the parent of a child with autism spectrum disorder (ASD), there is never quite a normal. I am Caleb's mom.

I use the phrase to settle my nerves after yet another tough day punctuated by running from class and screaming through the school hallways. Caleb, that is, is the one running and screaming. He is the one cursing at teachers and group home staff, putting holes in walls. His actions are predicated upon being told "no" while he is overstimulated. The combination is not good. I compartmentalize my frustration with a flat response, going into a zone of not giving a shit because I simply do not have anything to give. I've been down this path too many times, I have tried to figure out too many times, why did he do the fool yet again? I am just tired. I don't give a shit. I am Caleb's mom.

I say these words in response to interactions with others who clearly demonstrate some signs of being on the spectrum. In these instances, the phrase serves as reassurance of my assessments of others, because after what I have experienced, I know high anxiety, obsessive-compulsive disorder (OCD), repetitive behaviors, mechanical speech patterns, and overstimulation when I see it. I am Caleb's mom.

I say these words when I enviously listen to other parents highlighting the teenage feats of their wonder children. Their children are learning to drive. Their children are traveling to Europe for internships. Their children are taking dance lessons, participating in dance recitals. Their children are scoring game-winning touchdowns, home runs, and goals. Their children have a level of independence and maturity I can only hope for my own. I covet even the most inane semblances of normalcy in these parents' and children's lives. They have no idea how fortunate they are that they are not Caleb's mom, with autism seeping into every decision, action, or thought of him.

I remind myself that I am Caleb's mom when I roam my house, feeling like life stopped for us when he turned 11. I cry as I walk through the house, looking at photographic reminders of the skinny, impulsive child who once lived with us. I've closed the door to his room, leaving it a scattered testament of his inability to organize his thoughts; furniture torn apart in his anxiety-fueled fits. The pissy mattress because he suddenly started peeing in the bed at night, caught in melatonin-induced REM sleep. The tears, the anger, the weariness, the flat affect, the not giving a shit.

Yet, I am Caleb's mom on those occasions when he advocates for himself. If it doesn't feel right, Caleb can sense an injustice. "Call my social worker. Call my mother. Call my grandmother." He knows who has his back. And he knows policies. He is quick to tell staff at his residence actual policies because he read the policy manual on his own when no one was looking.

I am Caleb's mom, the mom of a revolutionary young Black male. Caleb knows his history and has no problem teaching Black history to others, including school staff. As a second grader, he pointedly voiced his objection to learning a sanitized, whitewashed historical rendering of George Washington. No. Revolutionary Caleb told teachers and classmates that George Washington was a slave owner, emphasis on slave. I taught him that Black people matter in the present and the past. I want him to feel good about who he is. I taught him to watch the news and read with attention to the spaces where Black people are represented, and the frequent spaces in which we are not represented. I taught him to look at how we are represented in the media. I taught him names and lives of historic figures, winding through the intricate connections to modern-day racism, sexism, homophobia, and ableism. He listens. Learns. And teaches others. Yes, I am Caleb's mom.

I am mother to Caleb, the young man who loves God. He loves going to church with his grandmother, in the tradition of many Black sons in previous generations. Grandma's church is more subdued; they don't have loud drums, tambourines, and the organ blaring. He likes hearing me sing but cannot deal with my church's 2-hour service. Grandmommy's church allows him to spread across the pew, ask questions midservice, and, from time to time, interject his scriptural interpretations during the sermon. There are older people and a pastor who has kids like me, he tells me. He feels safe in church. Well fed. Special. I am Caleb's mom and he loves attending church.

I am Caleb's mom. I am the mother who made the agonizing decision to place her 14-year-old son into residential care. The decision is still, to this day, the hardest decision I have ever made. Initially, I felt as if autism won, took my son, and left our family defeated. But, with the encouragement of Caleb's service care coordinator, who had also been forced to make the same decision regarding her autistic son, I looked at the state of our family. We were not enough for Caleb. We, in this case, was our patched family social net of myself, my husband, my parents, my elderly godmother, and my sister. The onset of adolescence brought amplified behavioral challenges resulting in two mental health hospitalizations in an attempt to press the reset button on behaviors and meds. It took his service care coordinator to help me see that we're not equipped to manage his increasingly frequent perseverative fits, aggression, and elopements. Unpredictable behaviors and increasingly intense meltdowns became the norm, shifting us into a state of social isolation. Caleb needed around-the-clock supervision and our social net was frayed, depleted, depressed, and exhausted. I am Caleb's mom, and I felt like a failure.

The transition to the group home was much smoother than I anticipated and Caleb adjusted well and rather quickly to having more medical and social supports. The transition helped me realize that all was not lost with my parenting efforts, as Caleb began to draw upon skills imparted to him. I soon realized that he acquired foundational research skills. He conducts a good interview, as he knows how to pose critical questions. Caleb utilizes his ears, his strongest sense, to decipher key bits and pieces of information. His ear-hustling game is strong. More importantly, he knows how to listen for critical information on residential staff, school staff, and family. He accurately reports information to me in a timely manner. He proudly tells the residential staff that his ear-hustling skills are acquired from previous generations—his great-grandmother, his grandmother, and his mother. I am a researcher. And I am Caleb's mom.

I am mother to a sensitive young man who cares abundantly for others. His strong sense of empathy leads him to open doors, assist the elderly, and love little people. He speaks up for his housemate, a young man with no family visits. He worries about the young man's feelings and calls him brother. He begs his grandmother to send plastic animal toys to him and his housemate, as he wants the young man to feel loved. He wants to share the plentiful love of his family with a young man who seemingly has no one. He has a heart for the world, including the sex-trafficked women he wants to save as a caped crusader. I am Caleb's mom.

I am Caleb's mom when I worry daily about his safety. Is he safe? Will his behaviors lead him to trouble in stores? I thank God he has the protective presence of group home staff surrounding him daily. Yet it is not enough. Beyond the presence of God in his life, will any presence be able to guarantee him safety? Some mothers do not have the same worries. My fears are exponentially raised. He is a Black teenager. He is growing and, at 5 ft. 9 in., will continue to grow. He is not small. His favorite clothing item is his Syracuse Orange hoodie. Tamir Rice, playing with a toy gun. I remind him not to use the broom as an imaginary gun while playing outside. Trayvon Martin. The hoodie I often remind him to take off when he is in public. The hoodie that makes me feel guilty for stunting his individuality and level of comfort in his favorite article of clothes. For kids with ASD, clothes are a battle, given hypersensitivity to fabrics. The hoodie is warm and comforting with deep pockets. The hoodie that strikes fear in the hearts of White America. Trayvon Martin. The hoodie that symbolized the abiding hate and anxiety toward young Black males across the country. My fears interfere with his level of comfort, individuality, and sense of being. I am Caleb's mom. And I am scared for him.

Introduction

The idea for this book originated from my own experiences as a Black woman mothering a son with autism. Since my son's diagnosis over 20 years ago, I longed for a community of Black mothers who were experiencing similar challenges with family and the lack of culturally responsive services, who spoke the same language. I longed to be in community with other Black autism mothers who were grounded by their spirituality; mothers who prayed and had no problem laying praying hands on each other. These similarities create feelings of familiarity, comfort, and problem resolution within a community. I needed to see myself in others who looked like me with similar cultural values. I needed to see Black mothers who moved similarly through the world due to the combined hegemonic forces of race, class, gender, and autism. I also needed mothers with the scoop, that is, information on various school districts and autism-related resources. Most of all, I needed a group of women who inherently understood that educating Black children is a political act (Collins, 2000).

My efforts to connect with an autism community via the web were fruitless, primarily because I could not relate to mothers who quit their jobs and devoted their lives to autism. I worked full-time and my professional duties provided some outlet from my autism worries. I recall that while conversing with another autism parent, who happened to be a White woman, she questioned why I moved into my school district and advised me to "just sell your house and move to my district." She presumed the ease of moving to a suburban town with high-priced homes, well-manicured lawns, and an award-winning district would simply eradicate the problem of schooling my son. And the assumption was made that I could actually afford a move. Moreover, as a Black mother, I also had to consider how a move to "her district" would introduce the issue of being one of a handful of Black families. No thank you.

My son was diagnosed at a developmental center that helped families across a nine-county area. During visits to the developmental center, I would watch and listen to other parents. I was unnerved by the comparisons White parents made of their children, comparing verbal communication skills and bragging about school achievements. The autism spectrum is quite broad, with varying levels of social engagement, reciprocal language, repetitive behaviors, and difficulty forming and maintaining relationships (Seltzer et al., 2003). My son is highly verbal, enjoys political discourse and Black history, and functions with some degree of independence. Yet we keep a close watch on him due to unsafe behaviors, aggression, social miscues, tics, and repetitive behaviors due to high anxiety. The developmental center waiting room, however, felt like a separate assessment process, with White parents questioning my son's skill set, sharing their child's skill set, and making unsolicited comparisons.

I would also overhear conversations between White parents about various resources they were using to "cure" their children. I was particularly intrigued by families who could afford in-home therapeutic services. Parents chatted knowingly about such services, specific providers, and the convenience of in-home therapy. The more I listened, the more I realized that although our children had the same providers, my family was never told about where and how to access therapies or even autism support groups. Moreover, we attended the same developmental center, and yet I had never been told about the process of acquiring a service coordinator, an individual responsible for locating appropriate services and placements for my son. I soon came to realize that developmental center appointments were tantamount to bank trips, meaning the center served as a place of currency exchange. The currency in this instance was information pertaining to autism-related services.

I learned these steps much later when a sorority sister overheard my autism-related concerns at a sorority gathering. I opened up and shared our family's daily challenges dealing with my son's school, after-school care, and doctors. She lovingly and firmly responded, "Sis, you don't have to do this alone. It's too much for you to handle." What I did not realize was that she supervised the disability division for a nonprofit organization. By the next month, we were paired with a service coordinator. We then qualified for services that I never knew existed, including respite services and community-based social programming for autistic youth.

During this time frame, a colleague asked me to participate on an autism parental panel. I was eager to share about my experiences, my son's accomplishments, and daily life parenting a child with autism. While the other participants shared about successes with in-home therapies and support groups, I described the challenges of finding appropriate school placements for my son. In doing so, I described the intersections of race, class, gender, and disability, sharing how my socioeconomic status afforded me forms of social capital that other parents of color in my district did not have. I wanted the audience to consider the ways in which these categories of social status often determine knowledge of autism and access to therapeutic services. I found myself in a situation where the entire room fell silent, with one person who angrily stated, "Autism has nothing to do with race. You have no right to bring that up here." Apparently, the mention of race made audience members uncomfortable—people who a few minutes earlier were comfortable discussing service inequities. I politely shared, once again, how social determinants impact educational outcomes, yet the White woman was unyielding in her denial of my narrative, my life, my truth. She was unrelenting in her anger toward me discussing race and autism, clearly offended that I troubled the waters of her autism conceptualizations as exclusively White. That moment cemented my need to seek out a community of mothers who understood the intersections of race, class, gender, and autism.

I mention the search for community, as I realized I needed to create one for myself, as the national, regional, and local autism community did not reflect me. I needed a community where I did not have to explain my expressions and my need to have "the talk" about race with my son. I needed a community of people who looked like me. My efforts to create a community of Black mothers of sons with ASD led to a loose collective of BAMs (Black autism moms). I met some BAMs via my sorority network, while I met other BAMs by way of family who knew someone with a child who had autism. In one case, I met a mother at a conference 60 miles from home. We discovered our shared connection to autism through a conversation. I was struck when this woman shared, "You know, you are the first Black mother I've met who has a son with autism. This conversation is so needed." She too believed that she was the only one.

I met with BAMs for outings such as mall walking during the harsh winter. Coffee talk at a café. Midday lunches. These gatherings provided an outlet for us to share our frustrations in persuading school districts to recognize the personhood of our sons. We used the time to cry about how we worried about our sons' life trajectories. We strategized how to educate school staff, family, and church members on the particularities of ASD. Gradually, one mother knew another, who then introduced me to yet another mother. These mothers shared experiences, resources, and most importantly, a knowledge of resources. In a sense, we had to create a community of our own because, yet again, spaces that service people with disabilities fail to consider how disability intersects with race and other identity markers.

The term BAMs was fitting for several reasons. First, my son, during the stage of sorting out what autism means to him, questioned whether a teacher's decision was made due to his diagnosis. He questioned, "Momma, is it because I'm autistical?" It bothered me because it meant that he too noticed differentials in treatment by teachers. Yet I was impressed by his ability to name himself, to create his own word to describe autism, thus, the name stuck. I shared the name Black Autistical Mommas among my group who understood the empowerment of naming ourselves. The name was well received with laughter and approval, as the mothers appreciated the use of Black English Vernacular to describe us in our own terms (Botha et al., 2020). They appreciated the inclusion of momma, as it evoked culturally grounded feelings of home and the comfort of a mother's love. Finally, the mothers believed the name accurately alliterated and captured our resolve to fight for our sons.

Notes on How to Read the Book

There are ongoing debates within the broader autism research and practice communities regarding the use of person-first ("person with autism") or identity-first ("autistic person") language. Person-first proponents argue that their language emphasizes and prioritizes an individual's humanity and uniqueness over a disability label. Identity-first proponents counter by emphasizing that disability is an indivisible part of one's identity and, indeed, one's humanity that fosters autism acceptance; proponents of both sides believe terminology is key to autism acceptance (Botha et al., 2021; Lei et al., 2021; Vivanti, 2020).

The tension between the two positions is especially dichotomous when writing on autism, as authors may be encouraged by publishers or peer reviewers to use one term or the other—person with autism or autistic person. For example, editors of the *Journal of Autism and Developmental Disorders* were compelled to address the issue in an editorial response and encouraged authors to consider preferences of study participants and social contexts in determining language usage. The journal's associate editor Giacomo Vivanti (2020) clarifies the journal's stance on identity language: "We support the judicious use of person-first and identity-first language in our journal as appropriate for the context, taking into account the preferences of participants described in each study and, when these preferences are unknown, considering how different linguistic formulations relate to different historical agendas, priorities and experiences of different groups and individuals within the autism community" (p. 692). While I am mindful of the debate over person-first or identity-first language, it is tangential to this study on Black autism mothers. The dichotomous nature of autism terminology did not factor into their analysis of their sons' lives, nor did it frame their advocacy.

There is a deep irony in discussing autism nomenclature relative to Black autism mothers given their absence from and over-exclusion by autism researchers, clinicians, and advocates—the same groups engaged in the battle over identifying language. Black autism mothers, as this study demonstrates, found themselves largely located outside autism communities fighting for recognition. From the margins, Black autism mothers push for a similar recognition of their sons' personhood and identities at the nexus of race, class, gender, and autism.[1] Readers will find a combination of person-first and identity-first language throughout the book. This variation both reflects participants' linguistic choices and is an effort on my part, as a researcher and writer, to engage readers across the broader autism community.

It will be incumbent upon the reader to make some choices when reading this book, most notably with regard to my voice, focus, and purpose. In writing this book, I struggled with how to position the multiple facets of my identity across the text with regard to being a Black woman, a Black autism mother, and a scholar. I figured out how to include my experiences in pre-chapter vignettes, but I was faced with the larger issue of voice and the question regarding for whom this book is written. I had to think about my audience. I finally resolved that I must engage two primary audiences: Black families with children on the autism spectrum and autism service providers (inclusive of those in education, human services, and medicine). My rationale for doing so was simple: neither group tends to interact or be in community with the other. As I discuss across

---

1. For additional insights, autism advocate Jevon Okundaye, himself a Black autistic male, describes self-identifying as Black and autistic (Okundaye, 2021).

the book, a larger problem of marginalization of Black autism mothers exists within the autism research literature.

My hope is that the book bridges this long-standing divide, unapologetically speaks to the particularities of experiences of Black mothers raising sons on the autism spectrum, and connects with multiple audiences. First, the scholarly community, namely those who conduct research on autism, needs enriched understandings of how race, class, and gender intersect to impact Black mothers rearing sons on the autism spectrum. Medical professionals can no longer function as if White middle-class mothers are the norm upon which all things autism are based. The BAMs included in this study have much to say about how they have been invisibilized by autism medical and service providers. They speak to their relationships with their sons, highlighting challenges faced when advocating and in turn the specific forms of advocacy in which they engage. BAMs combined experiential knowledge with the autism literature, the same literature in which they are invisibilized. Their experiences and insights could do much to inform autism research, especially that which relates to family-based treatments and the ways in which autism-related information functions as cultural capital for White autism families.

For these reasons, the book takes on an academic tone as opposed to a how-to approach to mothering Black sons with autism. Scholarly references and an explanation of research methodology, theory, and research questions are included. I would be remiss to exclude these elements as a researcher, but particularly because as a Black female researcher, I am aware of how the work of Black scholars continues to be dismissed by arbitrarily shifting standards. I am also acutely aware that the autism research contains very few studies by Black scholars. And, as there continues to be a paradigmatic separation in autism research, I recognize the importance of detailing the value of qualitative work in the field, especially as it relates to the particularity of experiences faced by Black autism mothers. Thus, I encourage some readers to enter the book with the larger study context in mind, understanding that scholarly elements are needed to situate the study within the research literature.

I recognize that research citations, study methodology, and theory may not interest all readers, as some people may simply want to dive into the narratives of Black autism mothers. The narratives shared across the book are quite engaging, moving, humorous, and uplifting. The language is real, frank, and raw as BAMs, including myself, speak authentically about our experiences mothering Black males with autism. While some readers may focus exclusively on the BAMs' narratives that begin in chapter 3, I strongly encourage engagement with chapters 1 and 2, because those chapters foreground the study with a comprehensive overview of the research methods and participants. I do hope, however, that the twains of readers' interests will meet, with readers leveraging the book as a resource with autism professionals. Integrating the research and citing researchers and statistics when interacting with medical professionals will help them recognize the need for more culturally responsive practices. One size does not fit all in autism research and services, and thus I encourage readers to leverage the work for the benefit of advocacy by using the book to demonstrate that race, class, and gender are very much at play in the autism realm.

Chapter 1

Study Overview

For many parents, an initial autism diagnosis is the beginning of an uncertain journey fraught with questions regarding life outcomes, therapies, and schooling dilemmas. An initial autism diagnosis may also lead parents to question exactly what autism is. Autism spectrum disorder (ASD) is a neurodevelopment disorder characterized by repetitive behaviors, narrow interests, communication impairments, and impaired social interactions (Centers for Disease Control and Prevention [CDC], 2020; Montes & Halterman, 2011). Children and adults with autism may demonstrate a spectrum of communicative abilities ranging from verbal to nonverbal with challenges making and sustaining eye contact (Seltzer et al., 2003). Some individuals with autism display rigid behaviors with difficulty adapting to daily social changes (CDC, 2010). For families of children with autism, this characteristic often necessitates rigid scheduling of family routines, as variation in scheduling, for some children, can lead to behavioral meltdowns. Physically, some individuals with autism demonstrate clumsy or uncoordinated movements and may engage in repetitive movements, such as arm flapping or rocking. Some fixate on objects, specifically the mechanical functioning of objects, or repetitively spin objects (CDC, 2010). While there is no cure for autism, researchers note that as individuals develop into adulthood, some symptoms may decrease in intensity (Seltzer et al., 2003).

Research confirms an increase in the number of children diagnosed with ASD, with a marked increase between 2002 and 2010 (Baio et al., 2018). Specifically, the rate of children identified with autism remains high, with as many as one in 44 children identified as having autism, with boys

4 times as likely to be diagnosed (CDC, 2022). Findings from Baio et al. (2018) indicate a racial hierarchy in that White children are more likely than Black children to be identified with ASD; Latino children were less likely than White and Black children to be diagnosed with ASD. This data further articulates that Black and Latino children are evaluated and diagnosed at later ages than their White peers.

Despite the growth in the number of autism diagnoses across racial/ethnic populations in the US, the majority of the clinical and practitioner-based research literature on ASD utilizes White families and children, upon which interventions are based (Pierce et al., 2014; Tincani et al., 2009). The additional perspectives of Black families, can, for example, provide additional understandings of familial participation, enhance treatments, and improve outcomes for Black children with ASD, as the condition is not limited to White populations as once believed and still perpetuated throughout the research literature (Dyches et al., 2004; Hilton et al., 2010; Pierce et al., 2014).

Insights into Black family practices, particularly that of mothers, is critical to expanding considerations of why Black families receive later ASD diagnoses and receive ASD-related services at rates much lower than their White counterparts (Dyches et al., 2004; Mandell & Novak, 2005; Mandell et al., 2009). Finally, the perspectives of Black mothers directly challenges long-standing perceptions of autism mothering as the exclusive, albeit contested, domain of White mothers (Douglas, 2014; Mandell & Salzer, 2007). In the next section, I briefly examine how mothers have historically been situated as the cause of their children's autism, beginning with the labeling of autism mothers by medical practitioners and researchers as *refrigerator mothers*.

Refrigerator Mothers: Historical Representations of Autism Mothers

The field of autism was fundamentally shaped by the 1943 publication of Leo Kanner's germinal study "Autistic Disturbances of Affective Contact." The diagnostic of "early infantile autism" emerged from the study, which focused on 11 children with shared behavioral and communicative behavioral patterns. Kanner, an Austrian immigrant, was particularly interested in the lack of social engagement, impaired verbal communication, and physical rocking displayed by study participants. The study was also important because it not only established autism nomenclature and symptoms but also blamed mothers as the cause of autism (Douglas, 2013, 2014; Kanner, 1943). Kanner based his findings on observations of mothers of the original 11 children in his study, during which he believed mothers exhibited cold, refrigerator-like behaviors that prohibited healthy mother-child bonding (Douglas, 2014; Simpson, 2003).

While long-standing castigation of mothers for causing their children's autism can be traced back to Kanner's study, it is important to place such claims into a sociohistorical context. Kanner's work, as noted by Douglas (2014), emerged during the latter portion of World War II, during a time of shifting and unsettling social order. Women, who in the prewar years had primarily occupied domestic roles, now occupied public spaces in the workforce and higher education. As Douglas (2014) argues, these social factors surrounding women filtered into what amounts to Kanner's (1943) chastisement of the mothers in his study, as these women possessed college degrees and worked outside of the home. Kanner's blame of mothers was furthered by Bruno Bettelheim (1959, 1967), who elevated the use of *refrigerator mother* to describe his subjective observation of cold and detached maternal behaviors.

Moreover, as Douglas (2014) notes that in extending autism diagnostic and treatment work to the domestic realm, Kanner (1943) and Bettelheim (1959, 1967) predicated their critiques of refrigerator mothering on social norms of White middle-class mothering. She said, "The refrigerator mother was also an ironically privileged identity (and continues to be today), available only to mothers with temporal, bourgeois, Mother American or Western European mothers. She emerged as part—and perhaps as handmaiden to—the post–World War II reassertion of traditional gender roles and push of white middle-class mothers back into the home" (p. 104). Said otherwise, the refrigerator mother label, under the guise of scientific knowledge, served to send the message that White middle-class women risk harming their children if they opt out of social norms. An autism diagnosis was thus deemed the result of White middle-class women choosing to pursue higher education and employment outside the home (Douglas, 2014). Although Kanner later reversed his views of mothers as the cause of autism, switching instead to biological factors, the damage to White middle-class autism mothers was done and adversely positioned them in opposition to autism experts.

Conversely, Black autism mothers were omitted, overlooked, and invisibilized in the original research that resulted in the refrigerator mother label, as both Kanner and Bettelheim used only White middle-class families in their samples. The lack of racial diversity in their samples continues to be an issue today, leading autism researchers to publish research based upon the experiences of White middle-class families and furthering the conceptualization of autism as a White condition. For example, a Black mother in the 2003 documentary *Refrigerator Mothers* commented, as cited in Douglas (2014, p. 101), "According to my doctor, my son could not be autistic. I was not White. It was assumed that I was not educated and therefore he was labeled emotionally disturbed." The mother recognized the double entendre of exclusion by virtue of race and inclusion in the offensive label of refrigerator mother as availed only to White women.

White Warrior Autism Mothers

Given the blame placed upon White mothers and their labeling as refrigerator mothers by autism researchers and medical professionals, it stands to reason that White mothers developed a particular form of autism mothering to directly challenge the refrigerator mother label (Simpson, 2003). According to Chivers Yochim and Silva (2013), *warrior mothers* are middle-class White autism mothers who publicly wage warriorlike fights against systems to win service gains for their children. Warrior mothering stands in direct contrast to negative images of bad mothering associated with refrigerator mothers because the warrior mother demonstrates her "goodness" or the qualities of good mothering by her heightened level of autism advocacy, and her refusal to take no for an answer. Good mothers, such as autism warrior mothers, leverage cultural and social capital to maneuver through systemic red tape, demonstrating that they are knowledgeable about laws and required services. Under the model of autism warrior mothers, White mothers are the holders of knowledge of what is best for their children, including treatments, school placements, and community-based services (Angell & Solomon, 2017; Eyal & Hart, 2010). The inherent knowledge of warrior mothers is in direct opposition to autism mothers from previous generations in that their work contrasts, contradicts, and rarely intersects with that of medical professionals (Douglas, 2013). Autism warrior mothers approach the acquisition of services from an individualized transactional approach, placing emphasis on gains for her child versus collective gains of all families grappling with autism. In these individualized battles, warrior mothers are rewarded by medical providers and school systems with demanded services (Angell & Solomon, 2017; DeWolfe, 2015).

Images of White warrior autism mothers now proliferate social media through websites, Facebook, and Twitter (Chivers Yochim & Silva, 2013), with actor and comedian Jenny McCarthy as the leading face. In the early 2000s, McCarthy emerged as the face of warrior mothers, authoring books on autism mothering. McCarthy leveraged her celebrity to launch a platform focused on curing and preventing autism, specifically promoting warrior mothers' ability to heal their children. She became the face of the antivaccine movement by attributing the cause of autism to chemicals in vaccines, although this claim has been dismissed as unreliable and scientifically unsound (Chivers Yochim & Silva, 2013). McCarthy's claims of warrior mothers' ability to heal autism drew the ire of the medical community and served to highlight a schism on who possesses autism knowledge: warrior mothers or medical professionals.

McCarthy's popularity also speaks to discourses and imagery surrounding autism warrior mothers who have formulated identities and support groups across social media (Angell & Solomon, 2017). While warrior moms share knowledge via social media and support groups, what tends not to filter into the discourse are issues of race and class as it relates to familial supports and services. In their study of Los Angeles–based Latino autism parents, Angell and Solomon (2017) found that while participants attempted to utilize warrior mother advocacy strategies, their actions did not necessarily yield positive outcomes. Their findings thus highlight the presumption of race and class neutrality in the imagery of warrior mothers, leaving mothers of color invisibilized in the realm of autism advocacy, fueling the belief that mothers of color do not fit the tightly prescribed image of autism fighters (Angell & Solomon, 2017). And, due to the focus on White autism warrior mothers, Black autism mothers' conceptualizations of their mothering roles is under-researched.

Black Family Perspectives on Autism

Research on Black families of children with ASD highlights levels of distrust of medical providers and educational services, with Black parents believing behavioral and social supports do not meet their culturally based needs (Carr & Lord, 2012; Delgado Rivera & Rogers-Atkinson, 1997; Leininger, 1991; Leininger & McFarland, 2006). Interactions between Black parents and autism professionals may highlight long-standing tensions between Blacks and members of the medical community (Washington, 2006). Routine appointments may then be viewed as intrusive and an opportunity to judge Black parents, in particular lower-income parents, making them feel uneasy and subject to condemnation. For example, Sousa (2015) describes the surveillance of mothers of special needs children including judgments of the mother's advocacy and caring by service providers. Families in need of systemic assistance must submit themselves to the scrutinizing judgment of service providers in order to receive services. Such service-contingent judgments are filtered through cultural lenses, meaning providers' determinations are mitigated by perceptions of social class, race, and immigrant status (Alston & Turner, 1994; Gourdine et al., 2011; Morgan & Stahmer, 2020). As noted in Sousa's (2015) case study of maternal involvement and family income levels, low-income mothers also described strategies of engagement with their children's development, despite systemic and institutional rebuttals. Broader inclusion of families of color can serve to offer more detailed understandings of how race, class, gender, and culture intersect to shape outcomes of individuals with ASD.

The research literature examining the absence of Black families from ASD research often conflates race with culture (Ennis-Cole et al., 2013). It is important to note that culture is not synonymous with race but instead more narrowly represents a worldview or lenses by which families determine values, childrearing practices, and traditions (Brown & Rogers, 2003). King and Mitchell (1995) describe Black cultural ethos as a worldview emphasizing collectivism and as spiritual and holistic. Black culture affirms individual personhood while simultaneously respecting collective experiences, knowledge, and being. Communal values and orientations, along with spirituality, serve as a buffer for societal micro- and macroaggressions targeting Black lives by the larger society. A Black cultural ethos, according to King and Mitchell (1995), builds knowledge collectively through the spoken word, thus solidifying socially constructed knowledge.

The research on the impact of culture on ASD is relatively scant beyond that which explores the impact of race on age of diagnosis, classification of symptoms, and access to care (Mandell et al., 2009; Montes & Halterman, 2011). Pierce et al. (2014) conducted a literature review of three ASD journals examining the inclusion of race and ethnicity. The review yielded low results and limited descriptions of participants' race/ethnicity, with only 72% of journals featuring research that included race or ethnicity. The researchers further noted that studies that did include race/ethnicity provided limited details on participant recruitment and included small sample sizes that limited generalizability (Pierce et al., 2014). It should also be noted, however, that the existing literature largely does not distinguish between the implications of race and culture, meaning a treatment of them as two separate concepts is needed. Said otherwise, theories of expertise must account for the impact of culture; as Collins (2000) argues, culture undergirds knowledge production because it is situated knowledge. Such theories of expertise, within the current corpus of autism research, however, rarely account for social contexts including issues of race, class, and gender.

While shifts in autism research now recognize families as a valuable source of knowledge, such expertise still primarily relies upon studies of White families, namely those from middle- to upper-class backgrounds, and provides limited insights on socialization and adaptation to ASD within families of color (Connors & Donnellan, 1998; Dyches et al., 2004; Mandell & Salzer, 2007; Myers et al., 2009). The need for ASD research on families of color is further compounded by glaring discrepancies in access between White and Black families to diagnosis and interventions. Black families receive diagnosis at later ages, an average of 1.5 years behind their White peers (Mandell & Novak, 2005). Additionally, rates of misdiagnosis of Black children with ASD are higher than any other demographic group (Mandell & Novak, 2005). Thus, the combination of later diagnosis and higher rates of misdiagnosis impacts long-term outcomes for Black youth with ASD. For example, a longitudinal study of mental health and health care for young adults with ASD demonstrated that Blacks have higher rates of limited care (Roux et al., 2015). Black young adults with ASD are more likely to lack transitional services (including vocational programs) and experience higher rates of unemployment and poverty, (Roux et al., 2015; Shattuck et al., 2012). Such outcomes further necessitate research on Black families caring for children with ASD.

Finally, it is important to highlight some particularities of experience relevant to Black families at the intersection of race, class, gender, and autism. Said otherwise, the matrix of oppression and privilege for Black families may necessitate different types of familiar practices or mothering that are currently under-researched. For example, families of children with ASD may focus social skill development on safety strategies, particularly as it relates to instances of elopement (Solomon & Lawlor, 2013). Nearly half of all children with ASD wander from school and home, necessitating police involvement in a third of all elopement cases (Anderson et al., 2012). For Black families, however, the involvement of law enforcement in cases of elopement could compound already nebulous community–police relationships and national tensions around policing practices.

An examination of social skills strategies among Black families of children with ASD could provide insights on the intersection of race, class, gender, and disability within Black cultural communities, further expounding cultural ways of "taking care of one's own" (King, 2001; King, 2002; Morris, 1992; Pruchno et al., 1997). Burkett et al. (2015) explored culturally situated caregiving practices among Black families, looking specifically at how cultural care informs health care for Black children with ASD. For example, Burkett et al. (2015) and Burkett et al. (2016) highlighted Black families demonstrating care through watchful behaviors. While the families described ASD-related safety concerns, the study explored familiar protective behaviors in relation to health care settings. Parents in the study were aware and concerned about the intersections of race, disability, and gender. While research has documented significant differences in ASD diagnosis for Black children with ASD, there exists a need to better understand what happens within Black families post diagnosis (Ennis-Cole et al., 2013). Specifically, given the cultural implications racial injustice in the US has had upon Black family socialization practices, what do these practices entail among families of Black males with ASD?

Black Mothers and Sons

This study examines the relationships of Black mothers and sons with autism, specifically examining how Black mothers socialize their sons. I chose to focus on Black mothers and sons with autism for several reasons. First, the majority of Black children are currently raised in single-mother-headed households, according to the Casey Foundation's 2015 Kids Count Report. This fact coupled with societal positioning of mothers as primary caregivers provides the backdrop for this study. Second, Black mothers practice gender-specific childrearing practices, largely shaped and influenced by intersections of race, class, and gender (Boyd-Franklin & Franklin, 2000; Bush, 2004; Gantt & Greif, 2009; Mandara et al., 2010). For example, Collins notes that Black women socialize their children with safety in mind, with protective actions framed by marginalized positionality (2000). She explains that Black women have been in the American workforce since enslavement and, thus, subjugated to objectification, sexual abuse, and other hegemonic forms of oppression. Black women who worked in close proximity to White families or men socialized their daughters to protect them against workplace sexual abuse due to their own experiences in White-dominated spaces.

Similarly, Black mothers have long feared for the safety and survival of their sons, particularly in light of systems of oppression that serve to target and marginalize Black men (Alexander, 2010; Bush, 2000a, 2000b; Collins, 2000; King & Mitchell, 1995; Yancy et al., 2016). Historically, Black mothers feared threats to sons' physical, economic, and psychological well-being from those functioning under the auspices of law and forces outside the law (Alexander, 2010). The story of Emmett Till, a Chicago Black teen killed by White men after being falsely accused of making sexual advancements toward a White Mississippi store owner's wife, attests to the historically based fears Black women hold about their sons' safety. In the case of Till, the White perpetrators were never convicted, thus supporting long-held notions that justice is meted out quite differently for Whites involved in racial crimes toward Blacks.

The fears of Black mothers for the safety of Black male children have been further heightened by stereotypical portrayals of Black males as loathsome violent criminals who pose threats to the general public. According to Kunjufu (1985) and Noguera (2008), Black boys, in the minds of Whites, shift from innocuous boys to public menaces by age 9, when they begin to enter adolescence. The power of racialized imaging, for example, was used strategically to ignite race-based fears of White voters in the 1988 presidential election (King & Mitchell, 1995). More recently, examples abound of how racial profiling extends to the attire of Black men, criminalizing them, as demonstrated in the killing of Trayvon Martin, a Florida teen killed by an overzealous neighborhood watcher. Martin's killer, George Zimmerman, believed the teen's hoodie denoted a criminal presence (Yancy et al., 2016). He was subsequently acquitted of charges related to the killing of Martin.

Finally, Black mothers are aware that law enforcement interaction is not a matter of *if*, but a matter of *when* in the US. Black males including Tamir Rice, Michael Brown, and Philando Castile were killed by law enforcement despite being unarmed. Specifically, Black males are disproportionately killed by law enforcement across the country. According to the *Washington Post* tracker, in 2016, 963 people were killed by police; 222 Black men were among those killed. Black males were 3 times more likely to be killed by police than any other group. By 2021, 5 years after the *Post* began collecting data on police shootings, the newspaper reported that 1,636 Black males died by the hands of police nationally. The *Post* also highlighted that Black males represented 34% of unarmed individuals killed by police, a figure disproportionate to 6% of the US population. Additionally, the numbers do not account for those killed while in police custody or by means other than shootings. The dangers faced by Black males at the hands of law enforcement have been further punctuated by social media video postings of police interactions gone awry.

The criminalization of Black men also has far-reaching consequences with high rates of incarceration due to a variety of factors, including federal drug policies and the "school to prison" pipeline correlating school failure to imprisonment (Alexander, 2010; Green et al., 2006; National Association for the Advancement of Colored People [NAACP], 2016). Blacks are incarcerated 6 times more than Whites and now constitute over half the national incarcerated population, with over 1 million Blacks behind bars (NAACP, 2016). The majority of this population is Black males. Thus, Black mothers have ample reasons to be concerned about the safety and survival of their sons (Green et al., 2006; King & Mitchell, 1995).

Intersectionality Theory and Motherwork

Intersectionality is grounded in Black feminist theory, which honors Black women's intellectual tradition, validates their worldview, and describes how Black women collectively develop ways of knowing (Collins, 2000). The theory provides a framework to understand how power, privilege, and oppression are shaped by multiple forces. Collins and Bilge (2016), elaborating upon the theory, describe intersectionality as:

> A way of understanding and analyzing the complexity in the world, in people, and in human experiences. The events and conditions of social and political life and the self can seldom be understood as shaped by one factor. When it comes to social inequality, people's lives and the organization of power in a given society are better understood as being shaped not by a single axis of social division, be it race or gender or class, but by many axes that work together and influence each other. (p. 12)

Thus, intersectionality provides a means of examining how autism mothering is a politicized space in which mothers and autistic children are positioned within a complex matrix of power, privilege, and oppression impacting access and services.

Douglas (2014) elaborates on how intersectionality impacts autism mothering and describes it as a space complicated by perceptions of mothers' identity, agency, and authority: "[Intersectionality pushes one to] think anew about some of our most intimately experienced ways of being together—as mother and autistic child—as not simply natural, nor a straightforward matter of disability or maternal oppression, but as interpretive and political sites replete with lessons about power, difference, and forms of agency within late modern life" (p. 2). Intersectionality is needed to disrupt renderings of autism mothers as exclusively White and middle class, thereby invisiblizing the particularity of experiences faced by autism mothers of color. Said otherwise, the matrix of autism and mothering is not race neutral, with race serving as a key determinant of oppression and/or privilege (Douglas, 2014; Angell & Solomon, 2017). For example, at the matrix of autism mothering, White autism warrior mothers encounter "disability and maternal" oppression while simultaneously exercising political power and agency to the exclusion and marginalization of Black autism mothers. Thus, intersectionality illuminates how one group of mothers can denounce ableism, decry autism discrimination, and concomitantly center themselves as the essentialized authorities on autism mothering.

Intersectionality disrupts the one-size-fits-all narrative of autism mothering and speaks to why a study examining the experiences of Black autism mothers is needed. On the surface, middle-class mothers with health insurance and high levels of educational attainment should possess valuable forms of social capital needed to access and navigate social, behavioral, and health systems. A singular lens of class, however, does not account for the disparities in autism services received by Black families, as research examining Black autistic children's health outcomes attests to racial discrimination when pursuing critical autism services (Broder-Fingert et al., 2020; Constantino et al., 2020; Stahmer et al., 2019). Class and educational status do not buffer Black autism families from anti-Black racism in service delivery and access. Thus, intersectionality provides a means of understanding the complexities of power, privilege, and access at the matrix of intersecting identities for Black autism mothers (Annamma et al., 2013; Carastathis, 2014; Combahee River Collective, 1979; Crenshaw, 1991).

An examination of Black autism mothers' intersectionality also requires a framework to better conceptualize maternal approaches at the matrix of oppression. Collins (1994) conceptualizes motherwork as a political form of mothering situated in the sociopolitical contexts of Black life in America. She elaborates:

> Issues of survival, power and identity—these three themes form the bedrock of women of color's motherwork. The importance of working for the physical survival of children and community, the dialectical nature of power and powerlessness in structuring mothering patterns, and the significance of self-definition in constructing individual and collective racial identity reveals how racial ethnic women in the United States encounter and fashion motherwork. (p. 374)

Motherwork is concerned with the survival of Black children because their physical and socioemotional safety is at risk across oppressive systems in the US. Those engaged in motherwork do not see themselves as powerless but are instead driven by the need to protect Black children's self-worth and survival. Black mothers are empowered by resistance, determination, and an unwillingness to accept social injustices because they understand their children's fate is contingent upon their actions (Harry et al., 2005; Terhune, 2005). In the face of systemic oppression, motherwork's identity focus ensures that Black children have a sense of wholeness and know themselves. Black mothers understand that self-knowledge is tactical when countering pervasive negative imagery, adultification, and criminalization of Black children (Alexander, 2010; Dumas & Nelson, 2016; Heitzeg, 2016). Thus, motherwork provides a theoretical lens to analyze Black autism mothers' multisystem advocacy for the collective well-being of their sons given their position at the intersecting matrix of race, class, and gender.

Study Purpose

This study draws upon intersectionality theory to better understand how race, class, gender, and autism (functioning here as a disability), categories of primary social status, coalesce in the lives of individuals with ASD. In this study, perspectives of Black mothers are analyzed to better understand family-situated ASD practices through the lenses of race, class, gender, and disability. The perspectives of Black mothers, a largely invisibilized population in the ASD literature, were examined to better understand how race, class, gender, and disability intersect in their parenting practices (Collins, 1986; Dyches et al., 2004; Mandell & Salzer, 2007). Black mothers of sons with ASD provide a particular angle on intersectionality, given the historical and contemporary threats to the social, economic, and emotional well-being of Black males (Collins, 2000; King & Mitchell, 1995). The study posed the question: How do Black mothers of sons with ASD equip and prepare them to confront race, class, gender, and disability?

Study Methodology

The study employed a phenomenological strategy of inquiry to better understand the phenomena of being Black, female, and classed raising sons similarly labeled as Black, male, classed, and autistic. Qualitative methods lend themselves to better understanding how participating mothers describe and articulate the ways in which race, class, gender, and disability shape Black mothers' parenting practices of sons with ASD.

Study Participants

Participants included Black mothers from Western, Central, and Westchester County, New York. The remaining mothers hailed from different regions of the US, including Texas, Virginia, and North Carolina. The 14 participating mothers were recruited by a variety of strategies. First, I engaged mothers I knew through my social networks. I am a member of a historically Black sorority, and I used that network as well, as it provided local, regional, and national recruitment pools. My sorority sisters then reached out to members of other historically Black sororities for possible study participants. This process yielded the majority of study participants. The second recruitment strategy included identifying Black church congregations in Western and Central New York. I emailed and called churches from the largest Christian denominations, including African Methodist Episcopal (AME), Baptist, and Pentecostal. Announcements were placed in church bulletins with study details and my contact information. A third strategy utilized social media. I asked sorority sisters and friends, who I knew had large numbers of followers on Instagram, Twitter, and

Facebook, to post study details on their pages. I also created a Twitter account with the intent of recruiting participants.

Study participation was determined by a variety of criteria. First, participants were required to be Black women, with no limitations placed on ethnic identification. While I recognize that White women are mothers of Black sons with autism, the study focus was specifically on women who identified as Black. The standpoints of Black women present, as Collins (1986) argues, unique perspectives at the nexus of race, class, gender, and other common social indicators. Collins elaborates by saying: "Black women possess a unique standpoint on, or perspective of, their experiences and that there will be certain commonalities of perception shared by Black women as a group . . . living life as a Black woman may produce certain commonalities of outlook. In other words, Black feminist thought contains observations and interpretations about Afro-American womanhood that describe and explain different expressions of common themes" (p. 16). Thus, I was very purposeful in delineating participation to Black women who mother sons with autism. Participants included a representation of diasporic cultures, as some mothers identified as Caribbean, African, and Afro-Latino. A second criterion was mothering a Black son with ASD. Participants identified sons as having a spectrum of ASD diagnoses, as some mothers identified their sons' diagnosis as Asperger's, high functioning, or low functioning. I am aware that these terms may connote ableism to some readers, positioning autistic people along a continuum of normalcy (Botha et al., 2021). Participants' usage, however, is reflective of language used when they received their sons' initial diagnosis. BAMs' use of outdated autism descriptors may also reflect how Black mothers are over-excluded from autism communities. Participants also described comorbid conditions of attention-deficit hyperactivity disorder (ADHD), OCD, and Tourette's syndrome. Participants mothered sons who were verbal, nonverbal, and minimally verbal. BAMs' terminology may be at odds with the autism community but is also a reflection of how Black autism mothers are positioned as outsiders among autism researchers and service providers.

In seeking participants, I did not specify income levels, as I wanted a cross-section of Black mothers to determine how categories of primary status played out in their mothering of sons with ASD. The participant group was comprised of middle-class mothers, all of whom had education levels beyond high school; all were college educated with some holding graduate degrees including doctorates. Study criteria did not specify marital status, as my focus was exclusively upon the participating mothers. Most participating Black mothers, however, were married at the time of data collection. Study criteria also did not specify a religious preference for participants, although most professed Christian beliefs that they exercised in different ways and varying degrees. The fact that all study participants are educated, middle class, and Christian does not preclude diverse perspectives of Black women with multifaceted identities at these shared intersections. For example, participants identified as middle class but represented a broad income spectrum within that classification.

Data Collection Methods

This study utilized a variety of data collection methods in an effort to generate rich descriptive data. Prior to all interviews, participants were asked to complete a participant demographic form. The demographic form functioned as a means of organizing critical demographic details related to participants and their families. Participants were asked to provide a self-selected pseudonym for themselves and their son(s). Demographic questions ranged from age, occupation, number of children, and number of children with autism. The second section of the demographic form focused upon participants' son(s) with ASD. Questions posed covered: age of diagnosis, current age, ability to verbally communicate, additional medical conditions, and safety concerns.

Family constellation diagrams were distributed to participants at the same time as the demographic forms. The diagram was created to provide a visual representation of participants' familial constellations and community support systems for their son(s) with autism. The diagram is a bullseye with the child at the center. Participants were asked to indicate family and others who provide social supports for their sons by adding their names and descriptive titles reflecting the relational connection. Those with closer relationships to the son(s) were asked to be placed in proximity to the center of the bullseye. The diagram is situated in Afrocentric research methods (King & Mitchell, 1995) and acknowledges the communal nature of Black families, which includes fictive kin (Boyd-Franklin, 2003; Burkett et al., 2016; Burkett et al., 2015; Stack, 1974).

All participants completed individual interviews that took place at cafés, a classroom on a college campus, or an office. Four interviews occurred over the phone[1] due to distance and travel limitations. The interview protocol, overall, sought to better understand how BAMs make sense out of mothering Black males who happen to have autism. The protocol included questions focused on their sons' initial ASD diagnosis and their sons' personality and social challenges. Questions then shifted to focus upon mothers' perspectives on raising a Black male with ASD and their opinions on what ASD providers, educators, and law enforcement need to know in order to provide culturally responsive services. Specifically, I asked participants what and how they taught their sons given the intersection of race, class, gender, and autism. Mothers were also asked about family support systems and self-care. All individual interviews lasted 60 to 90 minutes and were professionally transcribed. While the initial research plan called for a small group conversation with BAMs assembled in one location, this proved daunting and did not occur due to scheduling.

Data Analysis

Several rounds of data analysis occurred, utilizing both manual coding and electronic coding by means of Atlas.ti qualitative analysis software. Data analysis began prior to the first interview by virtue of a priori coding then progressed to several rounds of open coding as data collection occurred (Saldana, 2016). While the analytical software allowed me to better view the progression of smaller codes to the formulation of larger codes, I ultimately utilized manual coding as a means of organizing BAMs' thoughts into categories. Once these categories were organized, I returned to individual transcripts to ensure the inclusion of BAMs' voices across categories. The process then resulted in study themes presented here as chapters.

On a more personal note, the process of data analysis also served as an analytical process for me. For example, when participating mothers cried, I felt their emotions, as I did when they expressed frustrations. The more I interviewed and communicated with the participating mothers, the more I realized that the process uncovered feelings and experiences I closely held and had only expressed to myself in writing, as journaling was a space to process my own thoughts. Journaling allowed me to make

---

1. Data collection began in 2017, when videoconferencing was not yet widely accessible. Thus, details on all participants' physical appearances were not available.

sense of being Black, a mother, classed, gendered, and raising a Black son with autism and led me to realize that I was simultaneously interviewing mothers and posing similar questions to myself. The "I am Caleb's mom" narratives that appear at the start of each chapter are those journal entries and they bring an autoethnographic element to the study. The refrain of being Caleb's mom developed organically as a pronouncement of my maternal pride and protectiveness. Readers will see the connections between my autoethnographic narratives and data from participating mothers. This organization creates a collective voice of Black mothers of sons with ASD, while including my own.

In the following chapter, participating Black autism mothers are introduced in detail to familiarize readers with the mothers and sons. My hope is that readers will connect with the contexts of BAMs' lives to gain a better understanding of mothering at the intersection of race, class, gender, and autism through the standpoint of BAMs. This intersection will be revisited across the chapters with regard to BAMs' process of seeking autism diagnosis for their sons and the resulting processes of accepting the diagnosis. The analysis presented then shifts to specifically consider how BAMs mother at the intersection of race, class, gender, and autism with regard to their fears, hopes, and long-term goals for their sons. In articulating long-term outcomes for their sons, however, BAMs employ discursive resistance when advocating for their sons in various social spaces, including schools and churches. I then delve into the advocacy of BAMs, specifically connecting the fight for dignity and resources with a larger mission. In doing so, mothers share advocacy strategies they breathe into their sons, specifically, holding high expectations for sons, despite autism. Finally, BAMs offer medical, educational, and human service providers' culturally responsive suggestions and strategies for serving Black autism families. I then conclude the book with suggestions for future research and practice for Black autism parents and those involved in providing autism services to Black autism families.

Chapter 2

The Making of Black Autism Mothers

After completing a full day's work, I did my usual picking Caleb up from daycare. These times were the highlight of my day: I was able to reconnect with Bookie Man, feed him, play with him, and just love on him. He was my world, my heart, my everything. As a divorced mother completing my doctorate, my child was my anchor and my reason for persevering. He was my sidekick—if you saw me, you saw him. Because I lived 3,000 miles away from my family, Caleb and I created our own family, a support system of other students and church members. I surrounded him with people who loved him dearly; folks who taught him manners, introduced him to various foods, and showered him with affection. I established a well-organized life for us where we could both thrive.

Lately, however, Caleb struggled in daycare, specifically going on a biting and hitting spree. I chalked this up to communication frustration and continued to work with him on developing American Sign Language (ASL) skills so he could use signs to communicate. The daycare center director, however, greeted me one day with a request to speak privately about Caleb's progress.

"Mrs. Dingus, you will need to make other arrangements for Caleb's daycare."

"Wait a minute. Are you actually dismissing him from the center?" I replied.

"Yes. This really isn't a fit for him."

"What the hell am I supposed to do? I am 3,000 miles from my closest relative. I am working on my doctorate. I have three jobs. You can't just throw this on my plate like this. I need some reasons why you are dismissing a 2-year-old from daycare!"

Clearly, she had thought about this conversation well in advance, because she had the rationale for dismissal well prepared. "Well, I have spoken to you about the biting. And, he hits. And he has a hard time moving to different activities across the day. And, he bit the goat at the petting zoo. And, his language isn't developing as quickly as his peers. Instead of saying, 'I'm hungry,' he says, 'I hun-gwy.' I can give you some references for other centers where he may be a better fit." I was caught totally off guard, but I fired back a response. "He's 2, he's supposed to pronounce hungry in that manner. And his peers are girls who develop faster than boys do. I do get that he is a prolific biter, but most kids go through that stage."

We continued back and forth for 10 additional minutes to no avail—he was summarily dismissed from the daycare center. I was totally caught off guard. Within minutes, the conversation had shifted from the daycare center's director calling me into her office detailing Caleb's developmental shortcomings, to now, he's being put out of a daycare. The decision was made with no formal assessment. This is daycare, not Harvard! Daycare!

I left the daycare "hot as fish grease," as my female family members used to say when their anger reached a critical point. I went home and fired off a letter written in protest and disgust for the center's decision. I criticized the director for starting the conspiracy early, that is, the conspiracy to destroy Black boys, as detailed in the book by the same title. Dr. Jawanza Kunjufu (1985) wrote about White educators' roles in the educational experiences of Black males, in particular, low graduation rates, high rates of suspension, high rates of special education referral, and the ascription of negativity to Black boys beginning in elementary school. My familiarity with the research literature on Black children in US schools further informed my views that Black boys are targeted and labeled. My dissertation research on Black teaching families also resonated with differences in how Black women teachers and White women teachers approached teaching Black boys. My participants emphasized advocacy, high expectations, and community involvement. Even my experiences as a high school English teacher fortified my belief in the "conspiracy." Now, as the mother of a Black boy, I was mortified that the conspiracy started so soon, at a mere 2 years old. The following days were a blur of trying to locate a new daycare and securing his spot. I prayed for answers and continued to be pissed about how the conspiracy was playing out already.

Needing another opinion, I called my cousin, Wanda, who was also completing her doctorate in the Atlanta region. We had visited her twice within a 1-year period, as I traveled to Atlanta for fellowship requirements and returned later in the year to collect dissertation data. I called Wanda because her area of expertise is early childhood psychology and she had experience doing preschool age assessments. Most of all, I needed to discuss the matter with a trusted family member who helped raise me.

I recounted the conversation with the daycare center director followed by my tirade of how we were encountering the conspiracy. In her usual calm and rational voice, Wanda shared something I was not prepared to hear. "Well, I did notice some changes in his behaviors between both times he was here in Atlanta. During the first visit he was more engaged, during the second, not so much."

She further explained how she noticed his fixation on one toy, his ability to focus on that toy an extended period of time, and, his inability to make or sustain eye contact. When I asked what I was looking at, she shared, "I think he has autism."

꙳

The beginning of my family's autism journey foregrounds the narratives of Black autism mothers who share this journey. This chapter provides an overview of study participants with brief descriptions of each BAM appearing in alphabetical order. I began the process of data collection during the spring of 2017, with a few promises of participation from Black autism mothers. Outside of a handful of BAMs, I held no preconceived ideas of who would ultimately participate in the study. As previously mentioned, the number of participants grew through social media and word of mouth until finally a total of 14 Black autism mothers were interviewed over the course of a year. Due to my use of social networks, including sorority connections, my participant pool did not reflect broad class and income variations. My use of social networks also yielded a participant pool of women with education ranging from some college to doctoral degrees. The majority of participants were married or partnered with fathers maintaining active roles in their sons' lives. Most participants were over 40 years old, with a few mothers in their 30s.

I asked the mothers to provide pseudonyms for themselves and their sons, with most participating mothers opting to use their sons' actual nicknames. It is also important to note that nicknaming represents a Black cultural practice that recognizes some aspect of a person's character, personality, and the family's relationship with the individual. Participating Black mothers opted to use sons' nicknames that captured families' endearment in names such as Papa Smurf or Poopy-Doo. Nicknames also embodied topics of expert knowledge held by participants' sons. Ginger's sons, Music Man and Cat Man, are examples of nicknames that reflect interests. Additional demographic details for each participating Black autism mother, including age, state of residence, occupation, marital status, son's name(s) and age, can be found in table 2.1.

Table 2.1. Study Participants

Participant's Name & Age (N = 14)	State	Participant's Occupation	Marital Status, Partner's Name	Son(s) with Autism Name & Age
Donelle Boston, 64	NC	Business management, retired	Married, Gerald	Bear, 31
Candi Charles, 47	NY	Higher education administrative assistant/FT master's student	Married, Alphonso	Pappas, 17
Marley Christian, 35	NY	Nonprofit operations director	Married, Skip	Poopy-Doo, 6
Karla Daniels, 45	NY	School social worker	Married, Kevin	Andrew, 11 Mikey, 6
Thelma Fox, 47	TX	Insurance sales & tax preparation	Partnered, Micah	Elijah, 14 Solomon, 7
Kendra Green, 40	NY	Pharmacist	Married, Kyle	Papa Smurf, 7 Lil Man, 7
Beverly Hughes, 50+	NY	Offender rehabilitation counselor/coordinator	Divorced	Marvelous, 16
Ginger Lawrence, 50+	VA	School administrator	Married, Larry	Cat Man, 28 Music Man, 26
Sarah Mitchell, 46	NY	Administrative assistant/special education teacher	Married, Silas	Dwayne, 12
Faith Murphy, 33	NY	School behavioral therapist	Married, Anthony	Fat Daddy, 7
Indigo Odum, 50+	NY	CEO, nonprofit human services agency	Married, Sharif	Poobie, 17
Michelle Priest, 52	NY	School social worker	Divorced	Sam, 17
Lisa Thompson, 50	NY	Higher education administrator	Married, Carlos	John, 16
Kiara Williams, 42	NY	Bank manager	Single	Johnathan, 11

Source: Author provided.

Participants shared demographic information via the study demographic form, which was intended to capture important contextual details of their lives. For example, BAMs were asked about their professions as some leveraged their professional knowledge and connections in advocacy efforts. Information germane to their marital status provided a fuller picture of BAMs' in-home supports and safety nets for their sons. Next, I introduce each BAM to readers along with a brief introduction of their son(s).

Participants and Descriptions

Donelle Boston, 64, North Carolina

I posted an announcement about the study in my church bulletin and initially did not receive any leads on potential participants because the study was mistakenly introduced as a class. Despite the confusion, a fellow choir member approached me a few weeks after the initial announcement and started asking me questions about the study. Our brief chat yielded a connection to her aunt, Donelle Boston, who reached out to me via telephone, indicating that she would be willing to participate in the study. Donelle resides in North Carolina, quite a distance away from her family and in-laws who reside in New York State. She and her husband have resided in North Carolina for the better part of 30 years, where she worked in business management. Donelle's husband pastored a church for years as well.

During our introductory telephone conversation, Donelle shared concerns that her 31-year-old son, Bear, might be too old for the study and disqualify her from participating. I reassured her that Bear's age would not disqualify her and was actually a benefit for the study, as I wanted mothers of older sons too. In my estimation, a broader spectrum across the ages of sons could yield a more comprehensive picture of BAMs from diagnosis, preadolescence, adolescence, and adulthood. Donelle could also speak to experiences regarding autism when the condition was not as highly recognized and publicized. Finally, her North Carolina residency brought yet another layer of geographic diversity to the study.

Bear currently works at a fast-food establishment, a job he has successfully held for 3 years with the assistance of a job coach. Donelle worries about Bear's long-term care and does not want the responsibility of care to fall upon her younger son who resides close by the family. Our interview focused intently upon this fear, along with examples of how

Donelle's faith has bolstered her in navigating the murky waters of autism services over her son's lifetime.

CANDI CHARLES, 47, NEW YORK

I first learned of Candi after an unfortunate incident, when her son Pappas, 17, was attacked by a White man during a cross-country race. The assault propelled Candi into the attention of the local, regional, and national press. Candi handled the traumatic situation with grace while forcing all parties involved to maintain a focus on Pappas. From afar, I marveled at how Candi sought justice for her son while maintaining a calm demeanor throughout all her media appearances, even when the wheels of justice stalled. I looked up Candi's address, wrote her a note of support, and included a copy of a letter I wrote to the district attorney in the city where the incident occurred. She returned the correspondence with a picture postcard of Pappas smiling while dressed in his cross-country track uniform. The situation led me to question how BAMs keep their sons safe, and how can we protect our sons from daily racial microaggressions? I kept the card in my office and looked at it often during the process of conceptualizing this book. In many ways, Candi served as an inspiration for this study, although she was not aware of her influence.

 I was finally introduced to Candi via a mutual friend who learned of my study. She immediately warmed to the idea of participating in the study as she too had an interest in reaching out to Black autism mothers. We texted often and established a meeting date where she welcomed me into her home. Candi provided an easy interview, meaning our interview lacked the formal stiffness of two strangers meeting and felt more like two Black women who had known each other for years. I appreciated her openness, vulnerability, and courageous love for Pappas expressed throughout our conversation. During our interview, I also had the opportunity to meet Pappas, a loving, bright-eyed, handsome young man who loves sneakers, like many other youths his age. Pappas has a very close relationship with his mother, who even runs alongside him during cross-country training.

MARLEY CHRISTIAN, 35 NEW YORK

In my capacity as a college professor, I lead professional leadership development sessions for the local chapter of a national nonprofit. I enjoy leading the group as it affords opportunities to interact with a variety of Black leaders from business, health care, education, and the nonprofit realm. In other words, I meet people outside my higher education comfort zone while being challenged to translate leadership practices across various sectors. During one of these sessions, I introduced myself to a new group of leaders and shared details of my life, including raising a son with autism. I then shared information about the book, which was under development at that time.

Immediately after my announcement, I received a note passed to the front of the room with a name and number of a class member who stated that she was interested in study participation. As we went around the room doing introductions, Marley introduced herself by sharing her professional role and marital status, and identified herself as the mother of a son with autism and a 2-year-old mini-me daughter. She immediately came up to me following the session and shared the difficulties experienced in attempting to meet other BAMs. Petite in stature with an Afro-framed face, Marley easily impressed me with her intellect, professional drive, deadpan humor, and high energy. Marley is also best described as a listener, as she was eager to learn about my experiences mothering a child with autism to gain a sense of future schooling and service decisions. Marley is the youngest study participant and is still admittedly settling into balancing motherhood, marriage, and career ambitions. She is currently working on her master's degree in strategic leadership, with the hopes of shifting into a nonprofit leadership role. Marley relies on her faith and church community for support, as her family is still struggling to understand autism.

Karla Daniels, 45, New York

Through my work as a doctoral dissertation chair and advisor, I often meet students out at their workplaces to facilitate our meetings based on their hectic schedules. While working with a student who happened to be an urban elementary principal, we would often meet at her school. She would show me around her building and spend time discussing the influx of students on the autism spectrum. One student who was recently transferred to her school was Andrew, the oldest son of Karla Daniels. Andrew was experiencing challenges transitioning to the new school and often spent time outside the classroom trying to regulate his senses and decompress from meltdowns. As a result, Karla frequented the school and regularly interacted with the principal. After learning Karla's story, I asked my student to connect us. We exchanged numbers and began communicating with each other for check-ins. I too was dealing with challenging autism-related behaviors and appreciated a listening ear of another Black mother. In addition to our phone chats, we texted and even did mall walks in the winter, our way of getting out the house, getting motivated for exercise, and staying positive.

Karla and her husband are parents to four sons, two of whom are her older stepsons. Just recently, their youngest son, Mikey, was also diagnosed with autism. Throughout our interview, Karla described differences in how ASD manifests in each of her sons and the abiding patience of her older stepsons with their younger brothers. Karla has a refreshing spirit, a warm smile, friendly face, and possesses an easygoing manner. She exudes positivity, optimism, and uses humor to describe the challenges of parenting two boys on the spectrum. Her spiritual life also provides a foundation for her family. A school social worker, Karla has dreams of furthering her education and pursuing a doctoral degree.

Thelma Fox, 47, Texas

I have known Thelma the longest out of all the BAMs participating in this study; we have known each other since high school and are in the same historically Black sorority. During our college years, we spent many carefree evenings at campus parties, dancing, laughing, but always reflecting upon the bigger picture of what the future held for us. Years later, we ventured on a journey together, for in a sense we grew into autism together, as our sons, who are close in age, were diagnosed just a short time apart.

At 5 ft. 11 in., Thelma is a force of nature with humor, unyielding faith, and a positive outlook on the world that translates into resilience. A natural saleswoman, Thelma works in the insurance industry doing sales. Fitness is a passion for her, so she created a second business leading fitness sessions with an emphasis on '70s and '80s soul and funk music. The past 2 years have proved challenging for Thelma, as she was diagnosed with Stage 4 breast cancer, shortly after relocating to Texas from Upstate New York with the children and their father. Ever optimistic, Thelma is now in remission and created a one-woman stage show to document her breast cancer healing journey. It is also important to note that during this period Thelma started and successfully completed her MBA.

Thelma is the mother of three sons; the oldest is now 21 years old and stationed overseas with the Air Force. Her middle child, Elijah, was diagnosed with autism shortly after his second birthday. Now 14 years old, Elijah is a tech-savvy teen who makes PowerPoint presentations for his little brother, Solomon. Elijah uses the presentations to teach what he deems are proper behaviors to his younger brother. Solomon is 7 years younger than Elijah and was recently diagnosed with autism. Prior to his diagnosis, Solomon was prone to curse-filled tirades, hitting, and spitting. The introduction of speech and occupational therapy has significantly decreased the number of rage-filled meltdowns. Thelma is currently separated from her sons' father, who maintains an active role in their lives with weekend visits and attendance at school meetings.

Kendra Green, 40, New York

Shortly after interviewing all the BAMs I knew, I hit a wall in identifying potential participants and needed to expand my outreach through snowball sampling. I needed to recruit more participants because I wanted to reach Black autism mothers outside my network to ensure data richness and saturation. I reached out to sorority sisters who maintained active Facebook profiles. Almost immediately, Kendra reached out to me in response to a Facebook posting. A native of the same city, I had never interacted with Kendra, although several mutual friends attended high school with her. From our initial conversation, I was struck by Kendra's intellect, in particular her grasp of the service "alphabet," that is, the language service providers utilize to describe various treatments, diagnostic exams, and autism services.

Once Kendra began to share personal demographics, I was greatly impressed by her ability to hold together the multiple facets of life, while still finding time to help other autism families. Kendra is the only Black woman in our region who owns and manages her own pharmacy, which she intentionally located in an inner-city neighborhood to provide easier access for low-income Black and Latino families. She is married and raising twin 7-year-old sons, Papa Smurf and Lil Man, both of whom have autism. Slight in frame, Kendra communicates in a thoughtful manner about her full plate managing the twins' behaviors, therapies, and medical needs, as Papa Smurf also has sickle cell disease.

With the assistance of her husband and brother who resides with her, Kendra remains poised while managing their health and behavioral concerns. Kendra is the lone study participant who is currently in a community-based support group. She is also involved in advocacy online, as she reaches out to ASD parents, particularly those who struggle with toileting issues. She merges professional and ASD knowledge, informing parents how to leverage benefits for costs associated with toileting needs.

Beverly Hughes, 50+, New York

My good friend who connected me with Candi also reached out to Beverly regarding my study. Beverly and I were introduced via text by a mutual friend who runs a gym where Beverly and her 16-year-old son, Marvelous, regularly attend cycling classes. Originally from New York City, Beverly relocated to a small rural community that is currently transitioning into a suburban bedroom community of the city where I reside. The move from New York City offered Beverly cheaper housing prices, as she was ultimately able to build a home from the ground up for her family. The move also allowed her better access to services in a much smaller school district.

Shortly after our introduction, we connected in the weeks before my self-imposed data collection cutoff date. We agreed to meet at a fast-food establishment near her home. Our initial meeting also provided the opportunity for me to meet Marvelous, a handsome, large, dark-skinned young man with a beautiful beaming smile. Marvelous is minimally verbal, however, he articulates his love for Beverly with constant hugs, kisses, caresses, and a willingness to share his milkshake. Beverly, a proud Dominicana, takes pride in Marvelous's appearance and described in detail his daily hygiene regimen, including brushing his teeth. At 6 ft. 4 in., approximately 275 lbs., Marvelous towers over his petite mother.

Ginger Lawrence, 50+, Virginia

I stay in touch with many of my former students. One day, shortly after commencement, a student texted me asking for clarification of my study topic. I shared the topic with her and she shared that the topic recently came to mind, and she had the perfect person for my study. She briefly described her niece who resides in Virginia and then agreed to share information regarding the study with her. Shortly thereafter, I received a text from Ginger in which she readily offered to participate in the study. A native of Virginia, Ginger holds a doctoral degree in school administration and has worked in education for over 30 years. Ginger describes her husband as a partner in raising sons Cat Man, 26, and Music Man, 24, both of whom are on the autism spectrum. Both sons were diagnosed around the same time, at ages 4 and 2, respectively.

Ginger noted that her professional experiences as an educator shaped and informed her approaches to ASD. She also described how her faith bolstered their family through difficult times, including social isolation. Ginger draws upon her ASD knowledge in other domains, specifically in her church, where she leads a ministry for special needs children. Both sons currently work with community advocacy agencies where they perform duties that include baking cookies and shredding valuable documents.

Sarah Mitchell, 46, New York

One need only mention autism to Sarah to gauge her heightened level of passion toward autism advocacy. Sarah easily shares her deliberateness in sharing ASD knowledge and services in her community. I have known Sarah for 10 years through professional networks, yet this research allowed me to see a completely different side of her. I learned about the level of her advocacy and her keen ability to maneuver in the nonprofit realm and through school district red tape, directly connecting the work of her nonprofit organization to classrooms in her community. Sarah is intentional in her efforts to train teachers to work with ASD students on STEM-related activities. Sarah returned to school to earn a master's degree in special education. She just recently accepted a full-time position as a classroom teacher, both decisions inspired by her son Dwayne.

Sarah has focused her life on raising two sons, one of whom has autism. Her 12-year-old son, Dwayne, was diagnosed at age 4 with autism. Dwayne's struggle to feel good about himself is Sarah's abiding concern about her son. The West Indian lilt in Sarah's voice rises when describing his social challenges, as his long-term happiness is paramount to her. She admits that balancing her needs with those of her children is challenging, but she recognizes the importance of self-care, especially given her status as a two-time cancer survivor. Conversely, Sarah strives to sustain a self-care regimen involving long walks, dinner dates with her husband, and getting her nails done to maintain her health and happiness. She is married to a former professional athlete and lives in Westchester County.

Faith Murphy, 33, New York

Five years ago, I began each September in my typical fashion, teaching research methods to a new cohort of students. As department chair, I typically meet students well in advance of their first class with me. For some reason, however, I did not meet Faith until she stepped into my classroom. I was immediately struck by her intellect and noticed how Faith moves quietly, yet confidently, through the world. With these qualities, she quickly became a leader among a cohort of leaders.

As she completed the program, Faith's life was filled with momentous occasions, including a wedding planned entirely by her sister and the purchase of a new home. Incidentally, her new home is located just down the street from me. On a few occasions, I noticed her little boy getting off the bus, met by Faith's husband, happily running into the house. When I shared with Faith that there are small roving packs of young boys on bikes and throwing footballs in the parklike median of our street, suggesting that there are plenty of playmates in the neighborhood, I remember her voice trailing off. In that moment I did not think much of the conversation until I later learned that her 7-year-old son, Fat Daddy, is on the autism spectrum. Diagnosed just prior to his second birthday, Fat Daddy is an active boy who uses facilitated communication. He is extremely close to Faith and her husband, both of whom attend school meetings and doctors' appointments together. Faith draws upon her professional knowledge and training as a district-level behavioral therapist when making educational decisions for Fat Daddy.

Indigo Odum, 50+, New York

Indigo was recommended for the study by a former student who lives and works with her in their Central New York community. I traveled and met Indigo at her office, where she serves as executive director of a well-known and highly respected community center. While I waited for our interview to begin, I toured the center and noted the colorful murals, happy children, parents, and new staff in the process of training. As a former community center kid, what struck me most was the energy within the facility, from the garden surrounding the parking lot, the newly added credit union, and the newly initiated staff. After waiting for Indigo to finish up a meeting, I was welcomed into her office. It was then that I understood the center's energy, as she described the various programs she started, including the newly opened credit union.

Confident, smart, and poised, Indigo wove humor and homespun wisdom across our conversation to describe her role of mother, wife, and community leader. Indigo and her husband are parents to a daughter in her early 20s, who recently relocated to a neighboring city. The couple's son, Poobie, was diagnosed with ASD at 4 years old. He is now a handsome

17-year-old who has a placement in general education classes. Poobie is a loner yet demonstrates some forms of independence. Standing 6 ft. 2 in., Indigo worries that his physical presence, along with being a young Black male, will impact his safety. Indigo and her husband have nurtured him to have clearly identified goals of attending community college and living on his own.

MICHELLE PRIEST, 52, NEW YORK

I met Michelle 10 years ago when she worked with my son as his paraprofessional. In her role as Caleb's paraprofessional, I had great trust in Michelle and never worried about him under her care. With a beautiful pecan brown face framed by dreadlocks, Michelle was down-to-earth, humorous, and warm in her interactions with my son. She nurtured him across the day yet held him accountable for his behaviors, encouraging him to do well academically and reach his highest behavioral goals. We lost touch, however, when he attended another school.

When the call for study participants was sent over Facebook and Twitter, Michelle and I reconnected again. The process of involving Michelle in the study revealed that there was so much about her that I did not know, specifically, that she too is a Black autism mother. Thus, her ability to work so well with Caleb—helping him make seamless transitions—now made sense as she brought her own experiences to the classroom. A divorced mom of two, Michelle moved from Brooklyn to Western New York in search of family support, a new start, and a more affordable setting. Her son Sam, whom she describes as a 17-year-old gentle giant, was diagnosed at 18 months old and maintains a close relationship with his mother, attending community meetings, festivals, and church with her. Based upon her experiences, Michelle has become known as an autism go-to mother in Black community circles, as she willingly shares autism-related information on service providers, therapies, care coordinators, and school districts.

LISA THOMPSON, 50, NEW YORK

I first met Lisa a few years ago at a conference for women of color in higher education. We first connected after learning we were sorority sisters, but I was equally drawn to Lisa due to her knowledge of the higher education landscape in her city. This was the basis of our post-conference conversation, and somehow we gradually drifted into discussing professional choices made due to family situations. We found ourselves at the familiar intersection of being Black mothers to sons with autism, yet, this time, Lisa realized that she was not standing alone. To my dismay, Lisa informed me that I was the first Black autism mother she had ever met.

Our conversation then slipped into the familiar terrain of autism without the added weight of explaining why the intersection is important, feeling judged, or questions regarding how the intersection impacts our sons. We spoke a familiar language of behavioral phases, tics, and the constant fight for services. We also bonded over shared humorous stories of our sons' new or continued ASD-related behaviors. Following the conference, we remained in contact with quick check-ins and brief emails just to say, "I am thinking of you" or "be good to yourself through the challenges of autism."

Lisa and her husband are the parents of three children. John is their youngest son, who was diagnosed at age 3. John is a large 16-year-old who loves nonstop eating and listening to '70s and '80s R&B music, especially Rick James and Michael Jackson. According to Lisa, these songs provide him comfort, although he perseverates and is known to yell "super freak" at inappropriate times. Lisa and her husband have created an in-home support system but she is largely responsible for coordinating John's activities. Lisa maintains an even exterior and calmly approaches the challenges of parenting John with great patience, creative solutions, and sustained advocacy.

Kiara Williams, 42, New York

Kiara is a fiercely independent young woman, who has risen through the corporate ranks in banking. Standing barely 5 ft., Kiara is outspoken, thoughtful, and communicates her interest with her large bright eyes. I first met Kiara when her son Johnathan was first diagnosed with autism. Kiara and I would bring both of our sons to sorority meetings, social gatherings, and step team practice, which allowed us opportunities to discuss his then-recent diagnosis. Jonathan was a small precocious boy who loved being surrounded by our sorority sisters, intrigued by our hair, nail polish, and smiles. He was always well mannered, played quietly, and listened intently to his mother's directives.

When Kiara and I sat down for the interview, it had been years since I last saw Johnathan. He grew into a handsome, slender, 11-year-old young man who was still very attentive to his mother. As a single mother, Kiara prioritized Johnathan's well-being in all facets of her life. Kiara has decided to hold off on discussing autism with Johnathan until he is slightly older and has the ability to understand what autism means. For now, she and Johnathan refer to autism-related behaviors as "superpowers" as a means of him establishing positive self-worth prior to learning about autism. Kiara has fashioned a life for them with church activities where she finds social, spiritual, and parenting support from her pastor and other congregants. Johnathan is also currently involved in children's theater and earned a starring role in his school's musical production last year.

Chapter Summary

Participating Black autism mothers represent a range of experiential autism knowledge, given their sons' ages and geographic locations. All participants in this study are college educated and employed with the exception of one retiree. The next chapter highlights the autism journey of Black autism mothers, from diagnosis through the process of acceptance and action. The chapter describes the ways in which BAMs gained knowledge of autism, disseminated autism knowledge with family, responded to familial resistance, and how they shifted to action.

Chapter 3

"Black Mommas Need Action Items"

During the time of Caleb's dismissal from daycare, I traveled to Georgia to conduct data collection. My close cousin, Wanda, who was finishing her doctoral studies in early childhood education, observed some physical changes in Caleb. She too noted speech patterns in my almost 3-year-old boy. She also noticed how difficult it was to understand his speech and how he flailed his hands. This behavior, known as stimming, was heightened by frustration. She made me attend to how he lined up cars as a form of play that engaged him for extended periods of time. Under my cousin's encouragement, I reluctantly began the road to diagnosis.

Upon my return to Seattle, I sought out a diagnosis from the school district, just as my cousin had instructed me to do. The plan was to get a diagnosis from the district and then take that diagnosis, upon my degree completion and relocation, to the new school district. She stressed that early intervention was essential for his speech and physical development. When I went to the school district for diagnosis, the staff initially spoke to me like I was stupid and did not possess the ability to process the information they shared. I was used to this dance, however, as for most of my professional life, I interacted with White people who struggled to comprehend that Black women can be smart, articulate, and college educated with clearly defined life goals. The dance was tiresome, and still is, but I put my frustration aside as I was there to battle for my baby. I had to figure out what was going on with him to gear up for whatever challenges faced him as a Black male moving through schools systems and society.

I spent the better part of 15 minutes explaining who I was, my educational level, my career aspirations, and that of my ex-husband, a medical professional in the area. It was almost as if the staff could not believe that an educated Black woman could appear with her son and request an evaluation. The conversation focused on the fact that I was completing a doctoral degree as opposed to my concern for Caleb. That bothered me deeply but per my usual experiences dealing with White school professionals, I attributed the amazement to ignorance. Despite my complaints, I realize that my interactions with the evaluators could have taken a different turn: How would they have treated me if I was not a highly educated, middle-class Black woman? Would I have then fulfilled any preconceived notions about intelligence or the ability to care for my son?

I received a diagnosis that hinted at autism, but I was left with the lingering question, what does the diagnosis of ASD mean for the quality of his life? As a Black boy, school is already hard enough to navigate. How will he manage? Where will he be placed? And will he be taught by teachers who understand him as a person versus yet another Black male thrown in special education? I was scared. But I pressed on because I am Caleb's mom.

∼

Although I did not know much about autism when I received Caleb's diagnosis, I soon realized that the diagnosis marked the beginning of my family's autism journey. The diagnosis was an immediate jolt to action because I desperately wanted my questions answered about long-term education, health, and social outcomes. Across this chapter, participating Black autism mothers describe their autism journeys, focusing specifically on the process of autism acceptance and actions taken following diagnosis. I was interested in exploring how BAMs processed their sons' diagnosis and how the news affected their family dynamics, as families must often make adjustments to support caregiving. Parental acceptance of autism has long-term implications on parents' relationships with their children, but also on parents' ability to advocate for their children. Understanding their children's behaviors in relation to autism is a critical component of parental advocacy, as medical providers, schools, and autism service providers must draw upon parental knowledge of their children to develop appropriate strategies and responses (Marchand et al., 2019). Parents' ability to accept the autism diagnosis is critical to their ability to work across medical, educational, and social services on their children's behalf (Lopez et al., 2018)

Overview of Autism Acceptance Models

Autism acceptance models provide a means of examining how parents respond over time to their child's diagnosis. Parents' first step entails noticing the signs of autism, or as in my case having individuals close to the child identify delayed or atypical developmental behaviors, including repetition, social interactions, language development, or lack of eye contact (Siller, Morgan, et al., 2013; Veness et al., 2012). This period is also marked by parents' willingness to categorize their child's behaviors as unusual and, in turn, report their concerns to their child's pediatrician, followed by full evaluations by psychiatrists, pediatric neurologists, or child psychologists specializing in autism (Wiggins et al., 2006). The timeline toward diagnosis is further exacerbated by the time involved in the pediatrician's confirmation or dismissal of the parents' concerns, secondary referrals, and gathering of information required for autism evaluations. Families can interact with four to five doctors on the road to autism diagnosis (Goin-Kochel et al., 2006; Wiggins et al., 2006). Additionally, some families pursue diagnosis through school district diagnostic teams inclusive of speech and occupational therapy evaluations (Siller, Reyes, et al., 2013).

The stages of grief and resolution are two prominent models used to understand parents' responses to ASD diagnosis[1] (Elder, 2013; Kübler-Ross, 1973; Lopez et al., 2018; Marvin & Pianta, 1996). The models portend that parents must work through a range of emotions with grief manifested across several stages. Elder (2013) argues that parents initially respond with denial as they begin to sort through how autism will change their lives. Denial is then followed by anger and even self-blame for the condition. The bargaining stage occurs when parents desperately seek out fads and alternative therapies in the hopes of curing their child. The lack of a cure, as Elder posits, leads parents into a depressive stage characterized by feelings of helplessness and sadness. Parents emerge from depression into the final acceptance stage, resolved to establish a new normal in light of their child's autism diagnosis.

A second model conceptualizes parental acceptance of autism as a long-term process of resolution. Marvin and Pianta (1996) argue that

---

1. I recognize that these models are critiqued as ableist, with Kübler-Ross's work connoting autism diagnosis as the death of a child. The models are used here, however, to challenge the continued use of these models, especially as it pertains to Black autism mothers.

parents shift through a series of emotions post diagnosis and recognize shifts in their own emotional state resulting from the diagnosis. In the next stage, parents realize they must shift beyond their initial state and suspend questioning why their child has autism. Once questioning ceases, parents settle upon a reconfiguration of their child in light of the autism diagnosis. Parents establish a new normal by attuning to their child's strengths, which then allows them to advocate from a strengths-based perspective. A balanced representation of their child occurs, with parents articulating the joys and difficulties of parenting a child with autism, resulting in the stage of resolution.

These models are useful in understanding parents' emotional responses to the autism diagnosis but are not without limitations, as existing models are based exclusively on White parents' experiences with autism acceptance (Lobar, 2014; Tarakeshwar & Pargament, 2001). The exclusion of families of color highlights the need for broader participant pools and cultural competence in autism research. Considerations of sociocultural contexts underscore how families live, understand, and approach autism caregiving. It stands to reason that if providers utilize such models to inform services and interactions, then families are likely to receive care that does not consider the sociocultural contexts of racially diverse families (King, 2002; Lopez et al., 2018).

Research has demonstrated how the collective orientations of families impact mothers' ability to fully accept their children's autism diagnosis. For example, Lopez et al. (2018) compared the post-diagnoses responses of Latinx and White women, with specific attention to extended family networks. Study findings illuminated similar feelings between both groups of mothers, however, Latinx mothers' responses were influenced by family members' acceptance and understanding of autism. The collective orientation of Latinx families provided the sociocultural context in which mothers sought support and assistance with caregiving. Due to limited understandings of autism among family members, the mothers reported blame, isolation, limited offers of caregiving, and minimization of the diagnosis. Thus, consideration of sociocultural contexts in acceptance models is important for autism service and medical providers when determining treatment and delivering services.

Finally, the focus on discrete stages in acceptance models is problematic because it minimizes the importance of *action*. When faced with the diagnosis of autism, as existing models posit, mothers actively move back and forth between stages, spurred by emotional and environmental triggers. For example, a mother may transition from denial to anger when confronted with hard choices regarding her child's care. The financial weight of associated treatment and educational costs could also trigger anger and frustration. I argue, instead, that the use of discrete stages misses a key point in mothers' reactions to the diagnosis—action. The emphasis on action acknowledges their emotions while accentuating how they responded with action.

In this chapter, I conceptualize the post-diagnosis movement as a journey during which Black autism mothers' actions respond to the diagnosis. BAMs' journey begins with acceptance, as they grapple with how autism further complicates raising Black boys. Similar to other mothers, BAMs experience uncertainty, frustration, loneliness, isolation, hope, and resolution. While stages of existing models illuminate similar feelings, discrete steps with a singular focus on emotions misses purposeful empowerment, determination, and strategy of BAMs in response to the diagnosis. BAMs' journeys situate their actions in a sociocultural context, with family, community, spirituality, and historical marginalization informing their actions.

In direct contrast to stages, *pictures of action* frame BAMs' responses to autism, simultaneously capturing emotions and actions. Pictures of action detail BAMs' journeys, providing perspectives on relationships, faith, and communal support. Additionally, pictures of action provide insights on actions taken to access and utilize autism knowledge to benefit their sons. Like faded photos in old photo albums, pictures of action of BAMs with older sons describe a time when autism was not widely recognized within Black families and community settings. These photos have worn edges from turning experiential pages, sometimes softly or harshly, across the years. Similarly, like today's selfies capture events in real time, exuding the energy and buzz of the moment, pictures of action of BAMs of younger sons capture mothering Black sons in an era of autism awareness and heightened racial tensions. Collectively, BAMs demonstrate how action offers a useful framework to understand mothers' responses to diagnosis and Black family dynamics.

Picture of Action: Acceptance in Action

Like many parents who receive an autism diagnosis, BAMs reflected upon the meaning of the diagnosis for their sons' long-term outcomes and their families. Post-diagnosis thoughts encompassed how autism would complicate the already heavy task of parenting Black males considering sociocultural and political contexts. Mothers are mindful of the joys and associated tribulations of rearing Black males in a society that produces deleterious outcomes for Black males. BAMs were already keenly aware of educational outcomes for Black males and the challenges of raising sons with autism. Thus, given the seriousness of rearing Black males combined with the diagnosis, BAMs did not linger on acceptance but shifted quickly to action. This is not to say that BAMs handled the news devoid of emotion, because they experienced sadness and disappointment, as the diagnosis dramatically shifted their lives. The diagnosis also shaped how BAMs thought about their sons' futures. They realized their long-term hopes and dreams would require adjustments.

Participants in this study are college-educated Black women, some of whom hold positions in school districts or social services agencies. I recognize that these BAMs' educational attainment and professional status afforded opportunities that mothers with lower educational attainment and income levels most likely would not have access to. Thus, some BAMs entered the diagnosis process with the understanding that the outcome was autism. Ginger believed her work as a school administrator equipped her "with the tools" to recognize that her sons, Cat Man and Music Man, were not meeting developmental milestones. Michelle worked as a school social worker before serving as a substitute one-to-one aide in special education classrooms, a move that allowed her flexibility to care for Sam. She explained that shortly after his first birthday, Sam lost communication skills:

> I noticed that some of the language that he had at 16 months and 18 months, he started to lose it. Songs we used to sing and connections we used to have, he wasn't using that language anymore. He was staring out of the window, becoming more disengaged with me and with dad and just with the surroundings and that was unusual because he was always very connected to us. I noticed that and it was about 18, 19 months.

Michelle recognized the signs and immediately followed up with early intervention through her son's school district.

Faith holds a doctorate in education and works as a school psychologist in an outer ring suburban school district. Fat Daddy's diagnosis did not surprise Faith as she stated, "I was already leaning towards thinking something was going on, that was kind of a little more prepared for hearing them say that he was diagnosed with autism." She engaged in the diagnostic process with some idea that her child could emerge with an ASD diagnosis. Her professional training and knowledge of autism prepared her for the diagnosis while providing a larger sense of what autism actually entails in a school setting.

Even among mothers who worked in fields outside of education, early signs of autism were hard to ignore. Marley, for example, noticed that her son, Poopy-Doo, 6 years old, displayed behaviors that proved troubling and inappropriate for specific social situations. Poopy-Doo's diagnosis began with speech therapy for a speech impediment and development of his reciprocal conversation skills, as he did not engage in back-and-forth conversations. Marley then recalled how an incident during a Halloween outing to a corn maze caused him to "spaz out." Shortly thereafter, she began to assemble the pieces of his behaviors by documenting his behavioral triggers and other relative details. Her perceptive efforts resulted in Poopy-Doo receiving early intervention services (speech and occupational therapy) through a developmental center because of her advocacy. She described her experiences:

> But it was definitely difficult to learn that I was going to have to change how I was raising my son, in order to make sure he was as prepared as he can be for dealing with life. Initially timid, I think I feel like we are a little more empowered at this point, and definitely not as disappointed as we initially were after hearing the diagnosis. I think now it's more of an understanding of, just, things will be different, and we'll figure out a way to make it work for our family.

The "adjustments" Marley referred to were shared across BAMs, as their post-diagnosis actions were influenced by a realization that autism would further complicate their sons' life outcomes. Thus, BAMS were not exclusively dealing with the autism diagnosis and managing associated feelings; they had to reframe what it means to raise a Black boy with autism.

BAMs were keenly aware of the contested presence of Black males in US society and used the post-diagnosis period to strategize the health and safety of their sons (Allen & White-Smith, 2018; Bush, 2004; Dottolo & Stewart, 2008). Michelle recognized that autism is an inseparable part of Sam's identity and how he is perceived by society. She described how it compounded her concerns of raising a son and commented, "I think as a Black mom I had that in my mind that I don't just have a child with a disability. I have a Black male who the world already may think that he's coming to the table with less, so I right away want to show them what he's coming to the table with." Faith similarly shared her apprehensions of raising a Black male with autism by stating, "It was definitely disheartening knowing that my child was going to have a whole lot of different challenges to face, already being a Black male, now he's going to have this additional component to him that's going to make navigating the world that much more difficult for him."

BAMs provide much-needed sociocultural pictures of autism diagnosis, as Black mothers in the historic and contemporary sense "make the personal political" (Abdullah, 2012, p. 60). Participants recognized the ways in which the political holds implications for Black autism mothers, particularly in light of how society treats Black children. For example, Indigo, a CEO of a human services agency, approached her son's autism symptoms through a political lens: "I recognized that at 2, 2 and a half, almost 3, I couldn't discern a word he was saying to me. I said 'Okay Indigo, get over your stuff. Let's see what's going on.' I had to get over my stuff. It's not about you." The "stuff" she refers to was an awareness of how Black boys fare in public schooling.

Given her background in social services and experiences at a community agency, Indigo, who described herself as an activist, was cognizant of how disproportionate special education placements contributed to high rates of Black male incarceration (Alexander, 2010; McDonald, 1997). She received her son's diagnosis with concerns regarding the marginalization of Black boys in schools and approached the diagnosis with a critical eye:

> When he was initially assessed, the social activist in me was speaking up. I said, "Okay, the social activist has to bow down to the mother . . . the mother has to find out what's going on with your son." But with the initial diagnosis and people of color, Black people in particular, it's like the ADHD time in our community when everybody was being diagnosed with ADHD and put on medication. Some kids need medication, but we'll always feel like we're over-prescribed, over-diagnosed, over-analyzed, over-assessed.

Indigo provides an example of how sociocultural and political contexts factor into Black mothers' interpretations of autism diagnosis. She drew upon the experiences of Black men in her immediate community and beyond when considering how the *label* of autism held implications for her son's long-term outcomes. As Indigo highlights, BAMs recognized the deleterious impact of labels on Black males: labels that translate into social marginalization, castigation, and incarceration. BAMs knew that their sons' autism diagnosis necessitated a reconfiguration of their mothering roles because their sons' futures depended upon their actions.

Across all participants, the diagnosis awakened a fighting spirit resulting in the development of action plans, which in some ways served as a distraction from the emotions and stress of the diagnosis. BAMs shed tears and experienced a bevy of emotions but reconciled these feelings through action. As Marley eloquently stated, "Black mommas need action items" because the diagnosis necessitated movement. Describing her days immediately following Poopy-Doo's diagnosis, she commented, "I'm done crying. How am I going to figure it? What's the plan? I've cried these tears, now what? Give me a real plan. I need real, because Black mommas need action items. We got to take some stuff and we have to be able to say then what?"

BAMs collectively responded to the "then what" through political and socially informed actions as demonstrated in pictures of action, which further frame their autism journeys. Purposeful action leveraged autism knowledge and underscored BAMs' approaches to autism.

Picture of Action: Strategizing the Autism Learning Curve

As BAMs strategized next steps following their sons' diagnosis, they recognized how their actions are shaped by knowledge. The diagnosis of autism, for many parents, ignites a thirst for autism knowledge related to services, schooling, health, and long-term outcomes (Osborn & Reed, 2008). BAMs recognized that their sons' futures were contingent upon familiarity with autism behaviors, treatment trends, and laws. While some mothers recognized autism symptoms due to their professional backgrounds, other BAMs held limited knowledge of autism. Both groups of BAMs, however, actively strategized on how best to overcome the learning curve of autism, while they simultaneously developed autism expertise as mothers (Eyal & Hart, 2010; Jacobs et al., 2011). Similar to Latina mothers in the Lopez et al. study (2018) who became experts through mothering, BAMs described an autism learning curve that, for most participants, began with a search for relevant autism information. Study participant Candi had limited awareness of autism prior to her son's diagnosis. She shared,

> The only thing I really knew about it was the hand flapping. I didn't even know about the language barrier, that there could be no communication. I really only knew the hand flapping, and that's the only reason why I thought of it. I wanted to really know what it was. I didn't care if he was deaf or he was mute. Whatever it was, I needed to know what it was, so I could know what to do. I didn't want him to have anything, but I knew whatever it was, I couldn't help him unless I knew what it was.

Candi quickly realized the steep learning curve she faced forced her to learn about autism terminology, behavioral descriptors, and interventions. ASD knowledge also encompasses familiarity of ASD specialists, programs, resources, and treatment trends.

The curve can be steep, particularly if one begins with online searches and social media, as the sheer amount of information can overwhelm mothers new to the diagnosis. Candi took a different course of action by curating readings on adulthood. Utilizing an intentional backward design, she attended to life outcomes and used the readings to conceptualize future possibilities for her son Pappas. Candi elaborated on why she approached the literature with end goals in mind:

> I got him evaluated. Then I started doing a lot of reading. I went on the internet. I started reading books. But the funny thing was, I wasn't reading about what to expect as a kid. I really just wanted to know, "Oh, my God, what's going to happen to him when he's an adult?" So I started researching adults with autism, and I found a book . . . the guy explains about his language. He started out like Pappas, and how he saw language in colors and music. And I was like, "Oh, okay." So as I read the adult stuff, I just wanted to know, well, can he go to college? Will he go to high school? Will he learn to drive? All of this stuff, and that was what I was looking for.

The strategy was a means of enhancing her autism knowledge but also allowed her to maintain a hopeful outlook on Pappas's future and engage in purposeful action.

Michelle also described how the quest for autism knowledge was driven by the need to better understand her son. Countless trips to the public library and endless hours spent at Barnes & Noble bookstore provided Michelle with autism knowledge and insights needed to advocate for Sam. She explained this portion of the post-diagnosis period by commenting, "I began my journey into learning any and everything I could about autism in general and about him specifically; about how he ticked. How he played. How he operated. I threw myself into learning whatever I could because I want to give him the best shot." The "best shot," as Michelle highlighted, meant learning the autism lexicon quickly, as BAMs were expected to be immersed in the language of autism shortly after diagnosis. For example, Kendra described arriving at the special education table following her twin boys' diagnosis. Her comments illuminate the steepness of the learning curve as mothers acquire autism terminology while simultaneously advocating. She recalled, "The first meeting was an alphabet soup with providers using terms that were foreign to me," and added, "[It] took me a long time but I got it. I remember going to the first meeting and they're like rambling them off or something. It felt like I was in a foreign language. You know like, 1 x 30. I'm like, 'What?' Like, what the hell. One time 60, one small group with one individual I'm just like, 'Ha-ha.' I'm like, 'English. You got to help me understand. This is foreign to me.'" While the mothers in this study demonstrated self-efficacy skills in actively seeking and asking for help, it is important to remember that Black children still lag behind their White peers in diagnosis and services (Dyches et al., 2004; Mandell & Novak, 2005; Mandell et al., 2009).

As noted by Indigo, BAMs understood that power is wielded through knowledge of autism, special education, and associated autism services. If they possessed knowledge of autism, their sons held a fighting chance, with BAMs utilizing information to maneuver through service roadblocks known to many Black autism families (Stahmer et al., 2019; Straiton & Sridhar, 2022). The combination of cultural knowledge coupled with BAMs' education levels and middle-class status afforded the wherewithal to seek and leverage autism knowledge (Marshall et al., 2018). Conversely, BAMs also recognized that despite being middle class, Black autism families are still subjected to bias that directly impacts access and availability of autism services (Durkin et al., 2017; Maye et al., 2022). Astute BAMs posed questions to the literature and service providers (Lopez et al., 2018). BAMs used critical questions to guide their reading and formulate plans, despite the lack of Black representation across the autism literature (Jones & Mandell, 2020; Steinbrenner et al., 2022). Furthermore, BAMs formulated life plans utilizing literature in which Black mothers' voices are invisibilized, with the experiences of White mothers as prevalent voices. Despite such glaring absences, BAMs conveyed autism knowledge to their family, in an effort to counter ignorance, apprehension, and resistance.

Picture of Action: Helping Husbands and Partners Create a New Normal

Although this study focused specifically on Black autism mothers, the sociocultural contexts of BAMs' lives required attention to marriages and partners, as the majority of participants were married, while others were divorced or separated from their sons' fathers. Apart from a few fathers, participants described how their husbands and partners engaged with their children by sharing caregiving responsibilities and accompanying BAMs to appointments where they too advocated for their sons. BAMs' husbands actively participated in their sons' lives. The marriages and relationships, as described by BAMs, were impacted by autism in ways that are typically overlooked in the autism research literature: Black fathers' understanding of autism and their responses to the condition within the boundaries of marriages or partnerships (Hannon & Hannon, 2017; Hannon et al., 2018). The longevity of the BAMs' marriages speaks to how they developed resiliency and helped their husbands understand and configure their family unit to support their sons' ability to adjust to their sons' needs (Bayat, 2007).

The previous pictures of BAMs' actions provide insights on how they responded to the autism diagnosis with deliberate advocacy efforts. Similar to BAMs, fathers of children with autism must also adjust and process through the diagnosis, engaging in an orientation process of determining what the diagnosis means (Hannon & Hannon, 2017). The researchers describe orientation as a time when fathers adjust hopes of fatherhood to the reality of parenting a child with autism. Fathers process the diagnosis by figuring out what autism means, in relation to their conceptualizations of fatherhood pre-diagnosis and in relation to family and community members (Hannon & Hannon, 2017). Black fathers approach fatherhood with hopes and dreams of what their sons are to become, some of which are situated in socially constructed ideas of masculinity (Allen, 2016). Boyd et al. (2019) argue that fathers of children with disabilities cope and respond differently than mothers. Fathers may want to interact and engage with their children but are uncertain how to build relationships in light of the disability. A study of Black fathers of children with autism also noted that fathers grew into their roles, eventually demonstrating patience and protective instincts (Hannon et al., 2018). Indigo highlighted this point when she shared how families seek out her husband, Sharif, to help other fathers adjust to autism. "There are a lot of families and they speak to my husband more than anything, because he has a son. There are dads . . . I have a friend and a colleague who spoke to me in confidence. Their son is severely disabled, but he struggles with the relationship with his boy." Fathers must be willing to work with mothers on establishing the new normal (Elder, 2013).

Transitioning to a new normal also required BAMs to help their husbands move past disappointment and determine their caregiving roles. Faith described how the diagnosis caused her husband, Anthony, to turn inward as he came to grips with dashed dreams of Fat Daddy's future. She shared, "[He] had envisioned a different sort of outcome for his son. My husband was really into sports, and music. He thought that he was going to help his son become the next basketball star, and be all about playing football and basketball, like he did. I think he felt a sense of loss." Faith shared that she attempted to guide Anthony to a different level of understanding by outlining how the diagnosis was not a deathblow to the family; she stressed that they had to work collaboratively on Fat Daddy's behalf. She added, "We had some conversations about how things just will look differently for him. He may still end up being interested in doing some of those things; it's just a matter of helping him figure out how he can participate in some of those things." She believed that Fat Daddy could lead a full life, so long as the couple worked together to support him.

While BAMs explained autism and sought their husband's full engagement in caretaking, the process took time because husbands were stuck in denial. Sarah and her husband, Silas, present a picture of delayed acceptance as 4 years passed before Silas acknowledged Dwayne's diagnosis. Sarah initially engaged in the fight for services "like a single mother" and emphasized how she moved to action while he remained stuck in denial. "The first 4 years, my husband didn't acknowledge he had autism. I was doing this by myself. He didn't have children until later in life—you just have your first son and you have these dreams of what it's going to be. Then you find out that it ain't going to be like that. It's hard." She further described how the resistance hindered Silas's openness and ability to talk about autism as a couple and with family members. The necessary discourses surrounding Dwayne's behaviors and caretaking needs did not occur because her husband was not ready to speak openly about the diagnosis. She elaborated on this point: "I wasn't even allowed to talk about it with my family and his family more so. He hadn't really wrapped his arms around it. I put up with that because he *allowed* me to get services. If he hadn't *allowed* me to get services, that would have been World War III." The *allowance* of services spoke to the couple's relational dynamics, as strong-willed Sarah would not negotiate on services for Dwayne, despite his father's opposition to the diagnosis. Thus, while Silas may have struggled to accept the diagnosis, Sarah held firm and actively sought services not from a place of malice in response to her husband's denial, but because the services were in Dwayne's best interest. As a result, Sarah determined the best course of action with her husband was allowing him to come to terms with Dwayne's diagnosis on his own timeline. She explained, saying, "I let him be." By the time Dwayne turned 6 years old, he evolved, embraced autism, and now is a highly engaged father. Silas made changes to achieve a work-life balance and is now able to be mentally and physically present with Dwayne. Sarah expressed her gratitude that her husband is now more hands-on and elaborated, "I am blessed with a husband who will [come home, cook dinner, and do homework]. But there was a time when he couldn't do that because he worked in a serious corporate finance job."

Adjusting to autism did not come easy for some fathers; a few BAMs described how husbands resisted and even denied the diagnosis with detrimental impacts on marriages and fathers' relationships with their son. Michelle explained that Sam's diagnosis contributed to an irreparable rift with Kwame, her now ex-husband. While she immersed herself into action learning about autism, Sam's father wrestled with fatherhood in the context of autism.

> During that time I was with his dad, in and out of this relationship, because dad went through a lot of denial around the autism diagnosis. I think he thought he was going to outgrow it. My ex-husband is from Ghana, West Africa. Culturally these kinds of concepts like autism aren't really discussed in his culture. I think he thought, "Well, if I just don't talk about it maybe it will just go away." Pretty much I was on my own to learn about everything, talk to the teachers, go to the schools, go to all of the evaluations, digest all of the IEP [Individualized Educational Program] information, all of that.

She believes that rather than deal directly with their son's issues, he withdrew from them both.

Michelle's description of her ex-husband's withdrawal demonstrates how spouses can be in very different stages following an autism diagnosis. Processing autism information may not necessarily be the barrier to acceptance, however, as fathers of children with disabilities often struggle with the relational aspect of the diagnosis. Said otherwise, fathers grapple with how autism will impact the father-son bond given the ways in which autism manifests in communication and social interactions.

BAMs provided pictures of how Black families must balance work with autism caregiving. Indigo provided an example of how Black couples work collaboratively to support a child with autism. As her son Poobie grew older, the couple collaborated on how to best support his desire for greater independence, including walking home from school. The couple altered work schedules to ensure someone was home to greet Poobie at the conclusion of the school day. Indigo explained their hectic schedules: "Poobie gets home about 3:30 and my husband is there to greet him. That was the sacrifice in our marriage, but in the sense of my husband and I are passing ships. His father is there when he gets home from school. That was probably the best thing we could have done for him." The couple prioritized Poobie's needs and adjusted their roles based on his developmental needs.

The prioritization or centering of their sons' needs did impact BAMs' marriages, as caregiving took a toll (Tarakeshwar & Pargament, 2001). Lisa and Carlos were married for over 20 years and raised three sons, including John. Caregiving demands dictated their schedules, leaving Lisa wanting freedom to travel for leisure, respite, and relaxation. The family learned early on that traveling with John was stressful, as the temporary shift from daily patterns and routines caused him to melt down. "We used to go on these family vacations, and when John's ready to shut it down, he can shut down. Like, okay, this, it's over. We go ahead and shut it down. Or John has to eat every 2 hours or whatever it is, so there's no such thing." As a result, Lisa believed that she and Carlos both realized that couples getaways were not possible, as John required at least one parent present. Thus, recognizing the need for respite, they decided to alternate taking minivacations with John's siblings. For example, Lisa would take her other two sons on museum or aquarium excursions, while her husband stayed home with John. She explained the arrangement: "[Autism] even changes the nature of your relationship to where you don't . . . somebody always has to be hands on, so it's either me and the kids, and you and John, or it's me and John, and you and the other kids, but it's very rarely all of us together, and it's hardly ever husband and wife. So it has sort of changed that relationship, but it is what it is." While the couple resolved the vacation issue in a way that allowed John's siblings to vacation without worries of John's behaviors, the arrangement did not afford the couple time to work on their relationship. Lisa and her husband Carlos partnered on managing John's needs but acknowledged that it led to marital status quo, making it hard to think beyond the current situation.

BAMs also stressed to husbands that their presence was needed in their sons' lives to assist with developmental issues. They believed fathers could best convey information regarding puberty because fathers have firsthand knowledge of male anatomical changes. As a mother, Indigo preferred for her husband Sharif to have "man talks" with Poobie about hygiene and grooming. She humorously shared that her nose is particularly susceptible to adolescent odors leading to discussions of who will broach hygiene matters with Poobie. She said,

> He's got a father that's just squeamish. It's just interesting [with] developmental stuff, we're going to get through it, but the male stuff, I'm like, "Dude, you got to get over whatever . . . Come on man. He is not going to let me come in the shower and talk to him about his genitals, and the fact that I know the Wild Wild West is going on there. You got to get it tamed," but I know he's going to be like, "I can't have this conversation."

As the couple begrudgingly and jokingly strategized about who could best direct Poobie's hygiene, Indigo appreciated Sharif's constant presence in their lives and added, "My husband, I thank God for him. Poobie is who Poobie is, and he just interacts with him as, 'This is my son and this is who my son is.' A reminder of that repeatedly is not so much with strangers, but with family. You know that family are comfortable with him. He doesn't really have comfortable relationships with his cousins of his own age because he's different than them." Indigo highlights that parents play a critical role in how Black families treat and accept relatives with autism. She paints a picture of acceptance, with Poobie engaging in "comfortable relationships" with family. This picture, however, did not translate across all BAMs, some of whom described troubling family relationships, leading them to create community-based support systems.

Picture of Action: "Don't Demean What's Happening with My Son"

BAMs provided detailed pictures of how the challenges of raising children on the autism spectrum can prove daunting and overwhelming. Care requirements for children on the autism spectrum can intensify over time, as families manage behaviors, treatments, and demanding schedules (Dunn et al., 2001; Mandell & Salzer, 2007; Marshall et al., 2018; Sivberg, 2002). Familial caregiving can range from social and communicative supports to intense care duties of bathing, toileting, and idiosyncratic eating habits across their child's life span. Families juggle full schedules of appointments with doctors, mental health care providers, therapists, school staff, and other specialists. Due to ongoing care demands, parents often struggle to maintain marital relationships/partnerships and connections beyond immediate family.

Although Black families engage in collective orientations to childrearing, the presence of autism strained caregiving due to the intensity of needs. Families also struggled with caregiving because family members demonstrated varying levels of resistance, denial, and willingness to learn about autism. For example, while the majority of married participants indicated that husbands were involved in caregiving, BAMs still believed they bore the brunt of caregiving duties because they navigated autism services, appointments, and school-related matters. Mothers recognized the connections between their learning curves and the benefits of fully understanding how autism could shape not only the lives of sons but the family unit as a whole.

During the data collection process, I asked participants to complete a family constellation, a diagram depicting how families supported their sons, who are situated at the center. BAMs filled consecutive circles with names of individuals who provided care and those who regularly interacted with participants' sons. The constellations elicited rich but mixed responses from BAMs, some of whom described family members who were not supportive. Familial nonacceptance, limited caregiving, and harsh judgment of BAMs' parenting skills resound with Lopez et al.'s (2018) finding that Latinx families, despite the communal nature of families, may shun and judge mothers based upon the autism-related behaviors of their children.

Sarah had a similar experience with her in-laws, who challenged her parenting style, believing that her sons were undisciplined. During one incident, she described how family members misinterpreted Dwayne's autism-related behaviors as disrespectful and demonstrative of bad parenting on her part. According to Sarah, Dwayne has a strong sense of smell that contributes to sensory overload. While visiting with older relatives, his great-aunt's breath triggered a negative response, as children on the autism spectrum may struggle with social interchanges and can speak with no filters. Dwayne directly told the great-aunt that she had bad breath. The great-aunt and other family members immediately launched into blaming Sarah. While she was mortified, Sarah stood up for Dwayne and herself, admonishing family members to learn more about autism. She recalled telling them they could not handle raising a child with autism and added, "If they ever lived a year in my shoes, their asses would be in a mental institution."

The lack of family support, specifically that of in-laws, also surfaced during Faith's interview, with her description of how her mother-in-law approaches Fat Daddy's autism as a phase, in an attempt to dismiss or decrease the presence of autism in her grandson's life. Faith described one instance in which she tried to discuss the long-term impacts of autism on Fat Daddy. She shared how her mother-in-law insisted autism was a temporary condition, recalling, "[My mother-in-law] said, 'He'll grow out of it. He'll grow out it. He's just a slow talker. He'll grow out of it.' And we have constantly been telling her it's not as simple as he will grow out of something. This is a lifelong thing that he's going to have to figure out how to navigate the world with it. It's never a give it some time and it's gonna just get better kind of thing."

Faith further explained that her mother-in-law rationalizes autism as a set of distinct behaviors, like those demonstrated by her husband Anthony Sr., Faith's father-in-law, in a sense, citing his genetic makeup for Fat Daddy's autism. This notion led Faith to characterize her mother-in-law's actions as disrespectful, illogical, and ignorant. Despite continued efforts to explain autism, her mother-in-law did not "get it," which frustrated Faith. She responded to the continued resistance with patience and chose, instead, to emphasize Fat Daddy's personhood. "And it's like I wanna just say that's real ignorant and disrespectful of you but I have to be respectful of my mother-in-law. So I just say, 'That's probably not quite exactly how that works.' Try to just phrase it in a different way for her. But it's just really like, don't demean what's happening with my son because you don't understand." The family avoided Fat Daddy, who typically was not invited to his cousin's parties. She attributes the situation to the family's lack of autism awareness and a hesitancy attributed to his use of facilitated communication. "When he does get in his moods about being frustrated about something, he will just cry, or make noise or scream. They just don't know how to handle that. And so they just avoid having to deal with that by not watching him." She noted that breaks come primarily from her mother and sister, while her husband's family rarely, if ever, spend time with Fat Daddy.

Marley described her frustrations with family members who do not understand how autism impacts her son's life. Despite her parents' regular engagement with Poopy-Doo, Marley was frustrated by their refusal to maintain behavioral strategies she shared with them. Highly structured and rigid schedules reduced Poopy-Doo's anxiety, helping to reduce behavioral meltdowns. She humorously stated, "Grandparents need a beating," facetiously drawing upon culturally contested discipline for misbehavior because their noncompliance undermined her behavioral modification efforts. In order to counter family resistance, BAMs purposefully created community as a means of surrounding themselves, and their sons, in love, acceptance, and understanding. They harnessed Black communal traditions of extended family networks to fill the void of family support. BAMs refused to hide their sons but instead chose to engage in community settings, realizing that they needed social interactions in order to maintain their spirits. BAMs refused to be limited by their family's discomfort and sought to immerse their sons in community settings. They believed that exposure to events and people was a developmentally appropriate and necessary strategy.

When Kiara's son, Johnathan, was first diagnosed, she quickly learned the value of community on the autism journey. Shortly after the diagnosis, Kiara was introduced to an autism activist, a Black woman, who founded a small nonprofit focused on autism. The woman shared advice that continues to shape Kiara's life as she recalled receiving useful advice on the importance of accepting help. "You definitely cannot go through any of this without community. You can't. It's impossible, because isolation is a tool of the devil and when people are isolated from friends and community and people who can help them, it just becomes overwhelming." Thus, what participants lacked in family acceptance and understanding for their sons, they purposefully created in community settings. In doing so, participants demonstrated how BAMs proactively reframed mothering inclusive of community support.

Picture of Action: "All My Chips Are on God"

The research on families of children with autism and other disabilities points to religion as a coping strategy and outlines how families use religion to minimize stress (Tarakeshwar & Pargament, 2001). Religion can provide a space of solace, affirmation, and community. For purposes of this study, however, BAMs' culturally informed narratives made a clear distinction between religion and faith (Reed & Neville, 2014). Across their narratives, religion encompassed church-based activities: the physical spaces in which they socialized and experienced tensions with other churchgoers. BAMs' distinguished faith as an action—the actualization of their spirituality. Through their faith walks, BAMs demonstrate the faith tradition of Black women, which emphasizes a personal relationship with God, who serves as provider, counselor, healer, and a way-maker (Avent Harris et al., 2019; King, 2001). Furthermore, BAMs describe how their spiritual connections and beliefs were actualized through their parenting roles (Mattis, 2002; Reed & Neville, 2014).

Black women's faith walk takes into account the sociopolitical and cultural contexts of their lives and illuminates how their spirituality helps them frame the world. For example, BAMs believed that their faith shaped how they spoke of autism; the act of speaking negativity over their sons could unleash negative life outcomes. Negative thoughts were believed to manifest as negative speech, which then functioned as speaking negativity into existence. BAMs recognized the "power of the mouth" in actualizing negativity into their lives.

Kiara fiercely articulated the power to actualize negativity by advising other Black autism mothers to refrain from engaging in nihilistic discourses. She advised BAMs to recognize how power is manifested and offered encouragement:

> Find Jesus, find a community, and just pray over your child. Do not speak death over your child and even though what you see may not be what you want to see, keep pushing past it because your faith lies in the unseen. My life changed because of that. And even though now I don't know what [Johnathan] is going to be and I don't even want to speak it because I don't want to put him into something that God doesn't want him into, but I just speak the success.

She shared that she received a prophetic word of healing, saying, "All my chips are on God. I believe He can do it." The importance of positivity was further punctuated by the sociopolitical context of being Black and male in American schools, health care, and social systems that already hold negative expectations (Marchand et al., 2019). Mothers recognized they are raising sons in a society that already speaks negativity over Black males, thus, their faith was a means of countering low expectations with empowering words and actions.

The picture of action also captures BAMs' speaking positivity over themselves, as a means of empowerment and self-preservation. For example, Marley attributed her ability to bear the load of mothering two children, marriage, school, and career by crediting God, saying, "My Lord says, 'My yoke is easy, and His strength is sufficient.' He's made my burden light. These are the things so if I've asked for it, I have to find a way to stay positive. I can't allow negativity to interfere with this work that I'm doing because it's bigger than me; it's so much bigger than me. The only negativity I can allow in my life right now is a pregnancy test. I can't even, okay? I can't." Marley's testimony speaks to how Black women have historically turned to faith as a means of self-preservation and to provide a broader perspective on individual problems (Burkett et al., 2016; King, 2011; Rogers-Dulan & Blacher, 1995). Incidentally, her wittiness also speaks to the importance of humor, as the ability to laugh at oneself brings levity to even the most challenging circumstances.

The challenges of parenting two sons with autism might appear as a burden, but Ginger applied a spiritually situated outlook to her circumstances that allowed her to achieve peace of mind and comfort (Lopez et al., 2018; Marvin & Pianta, 1996; Mattis, 2002). Moreover, Ginger's faith allowed her to make meaning out of her circumstances of mothering two adult sons with autism, Cat Man and Music Man. She derived meaning through service to others and explained, "I give. I serve. That's the one thing you can do that keeps you from being depressed. Because there's always somebody with a need that you can meet. And my father and my mother told me that if you serve someone else, if you're always a blessing, you'll be blessed. So that's how I spend my time. And I'm blessed by serving others, and encouraging others, helping others." Faith, actualized through service, helped Ginger conceptualize her mothering as connected to a larger mission of helping others. Said otherwise, she believed her mothering duties were part of a larger service calling connected to her faith. Additionally, Ginger's own spirit was renewed, allowing her to persevere on the autism journey. Finally, BAMs counted on God to do the impossible or, in Sarah's case, to win the fight with her school district to cover the cost of private school placement for Dwayne. Districts are often reluctant to do so, because sending a high-needs student out of district comes at great expense. Districts must cover tuition, service, and transportation expenses associated with students' disabilities. Despite her district's reputation for denying out-of-district placements and countless numbers of people who discouraged her from pursuing the placement, Sarah's faith allowed her to remain optimistic as she said, "I don't believe in logic; I believe in God."

Picture of Action: "Make the Best Lemonade"

I would be remiss if a discussion of BAMs' emotional states and coping strategies were not included in the analysis. Doing so perpetuates the problematic trope of strong Black superwomen powering through overwhelming odds, problem solving for their families and communities. With strength, resilience, and resolve, Black superwomen prioritize the needs of others and sacrifice their health and wellness (Abrams et al., 2014; Woods-Giscombe, 2010). Black women deal with racial-gendered sociopolitical contexts where they are invisibilized, marginalized, and silenced. Cumulative stress produces deleterious health outcomes, including depression, high blood pressure, obesity, and heart ailments (Woods-Giscombe, 2010; Woods-Giscombe et al., 2019). BAMs provide pictures of action, yet underneath the appearance of unassailable strength, they maneuver through stress, self-doubt, and feelings of guilt. BAMs developed strategies of self-encouragement, positivity, and faith.

The emotional work of mothering a son with autism is documented in the research literature with a focus on maternal stress (Duerte et al., 2005; Dunn et al., 2001; Mandell & Salzer, 2007; Marshall et al., 2018; Sivberg, 2002). Similarly, research on Black mothers highlights resiliency as an essential factor in mothering children in light of racist and class-based systems of oppressions (Harry et al., 2005; Hill, 2001; King, 2001; King & Mitchell, 1995). BAMs in this study add much-needed perspectives on the emotional work Black mothers engage in to raise children, with attention to how they manage the feelings under the presumed veneer of strength.

Across study participants, BAMs experienced stress related to managing their sons' care, schedules, and behaviors, some of which included emotional meltdowns, high anxiety, repetition, biting, kicking, screaming, cursing, and elopement. For example, Lisa described how her son John is obsessed with food and eats compulsively. These behaviors have led to safety concerns with the stove, as he recently began turning up the flame on the stove to hurry the cooking process. In response to these safety concerns, she noted that being told "no" serves as a behavioral trigger, with little room for negotiation. She commented, "When he was little, I used to question, 'What is the difference between negotiating with John and negotiating with terrorists?' You can't negotiate with this kid." The resulting "test of wills" often left her frustrated, tired, and sad. Lisa shared how during those times, she often wondered what John's life would be like without autism and commented, "Sometimes it really makes me so sad, because I just wonder, what he would be? What kind of kid would he be? What kind of person would he be if he weren't autistic?"

Autism does not come with a how-to manual filled with proven methods that apply to all individuals on the autism spectrum. The difficult task of navigating care systems and other caregiving decisions caused some study participants to feel guilty with some second-guessing themselves. In retrospective moments, BAMs described how they reconciled feelings of guilt by invoking self-compassion. Michelle pinpointed an instance of feeling guilty about a decision she made involving Sam's diet. When the gluten-free diet craze among autism parents emerged, Michelle decided to try out the diet, to help Sam's sensory regulation. Over time, she realized the diet did not lead to sensory changes in Sam and that the high cost of gluten-free and organic foods prevented her from sticking to the diet. The decision also made her realize that she was depriving Sam of the one food he actually enjoyed eating—pasta. She followed up: "Mothers of children with disabilities, we have a whole other level of guilt because we're never sure. Are we doing the right thing?" In turn, she refrained from berating herself and resolved to go easier on herself.

It is troubling to think of how the cumulative effects of guilt and self-criticism weigh upon mothers of children with autism. Given the intensity of care required, it stands to reason that mothers will make decisions that leave them yearning for do-overs. The journey, however, does not often afford do-overs, and thus self-compassion functioned as a powerful means of self-preservation and maintaining some level of optimism. Elijah and Solomon's mother, Thelma, reflected on the power of maternal self-compassion and the importance of BAMs being kind to themselves. She said, "Don't be afraid to follow your gut or do whatever you have to do to ensure they have a fulfilling life. They only get one. They are deserving of a good quality life." Thus, BAMs understood that self-compassion was a much-needed form of self-care, a means of gentle self-reflection, which in turn allowed them to better care for their sons over the journey.

Self-compassion helped BAMs move forward with caregiving and advocacy, as opposed to being stuck in past actions. Michelle resolved years ago that she needed to be patient and compassionate with herself because it subsequently impacted her and Sam's relationship. She elucidated this point: "I learned a long time ago to give myself a break and forgive myself for not having perfection. I don't know if things would have been different. Maybe not. I also know things aren't that bad either. It took time. It took a lot of time for me to appreciate who he is, who I am, and what our lives are." Self-compassion also occurred when mothers asked their sons for forgiveness during episodes of lost patience, frustration, and fatigue. Work-life balance was a struggle for some participants, especially if they were the sole income source for their families. Michelle learned to ask her son for forgiveness, particularly during times she was physically unable to be by his side due to her work schedule. She and other BAMs realized self-compassion and the understanding of their sons was key to alleviating self-imposed guilt and freed them from the constant need for perfection. Self-compassion was essential to Ginger staying the course of mothering two sons with autism; she did the best she could with balancing constant care demands with her own needs. Maintaining a positive outlook despite the lemons life may give you was Ginger's approach to self-care and managing stress. She said, "There's more I would probably do for me, if I didn't have this situation. But because I do, then I do the best I can. I make the best lemonade you ever tasted."

Chapter Summary

The period leading up to and immediately following an autism diagnosis can trigger a variety of emotional responses in parents. Models representing stages of acceptance provide a means of understanding parental reactions and responses over time. Existing models, however, are predicated upon the experiences of White families, with White mothers' experiences centered. In doing so, autism parental acceptance models neglect the sociopolitical and cultural contexts in which families function. The models also fail to consider the underlying actions and decision-making process of parents as they navigate post diagnosis.

Black autism mothers in this study, instead, offer what I call pictures of action—detailed insights of action, movement, and momentum. The pictorial framework highlights post-diagnosis actions underscored by sociopolitical and cultural contexts that already stigmatize Black mothers and sons. BAMs were astutely aware that their actions, specifically overcoming the autism learning curve, directly correlated to their sons' long-term quality of life. BAMs also detailed how the autism diagnosis impacted relationships, with fathers initially struggling to understand how to parent their sons. As such, marital relationships were impacted, with a few BAMs highlighting how they, along with their husbands, adjusted schedules and sacrificed intimacy to collectively provide wraparound support for their sons. BAMs' accounts of marital challenges provide much-needed perspectives on how caregiving impacts Black couples.

Black mothers participating in this study also described the need to acclimate and educate family members about autism, autism-related behaviors, and the subsequent implications on their parenting approaches. Some detailed tenuous relationships with family members who denied, rationalized, or explained away the diagnosis. These responses placed an additional burden on BAMs, as some felt attacked and judged by family who disapproved of autism-related behaviors. This was especially stress inducing for BAMs, as Black mothers are already critiqued, penalized, and maligned (Abdullah, 2012). In response, savvy BAMs created community-based support systems in an effort to surround themselves and their sons with love and care. Familial lack of autism understanding furthered their resolve to fully engage their sons in social situations, as opposed to cloistering them.

The framework of action illuminated the stress Black women incur from caregiving and navigating family resistance. Black autism mothers looked to their Christian faith for peace, strength, and meaning-making, as they continuously sought spiritual consolation across the autism journey. Tapping into a Black faith tradition helped BAMs stay focused on caregiving because they trusted God for empowerment and answers (King, 2001). Participants countered negativity with their Christian faith and found renewed strength and hope. They connected positive outcomes for sons with the power of positive affirmations spoken over their sons. Positivity then extended to gentle and kind assessments of self, with BAMs determined to exercise forgiveness for accrued mothering mistakes. Given the challenges Black mothers already face coupled with those associated with autism, BAMs realized that they would make mistakes along the autism journey. Instead of being mired down with guilt, BAMs treated themselves gently and exercised self-compassion.

Chapter 4

Black Mothers at the Intersection of Race, Class, Gender, and Autism

The day was progressing well, or as well as a typical Saturday could progress. Perhaps it is my fault that I did not provide enough detail on our plans for the day, or maybe I just wanted to chill at home and unwind from a stressful week. I recall that Caleb became agitated because I told him no, a word that served to trigger perseverative behaviors and aggression. He began to fixate and his behaviors soon escalated with his voice rising to a high-pitched squeal, his face turning red, and the constant refrain of "I'm sorry, I'm sorry." My strategy for remaining calm and helping him gain homeostasis was to remove myself from the room, head upstairs, and return once I determined that he was calm enough to actually reason within the moment. I went upstairs for a few minutes and decided to use the opportunity to take a quick shower. I returned downstairs and, to my surprise, he was gone. He was in the wind.

I panicked, but somehow I managed to keep a cool head. I remembered the plan my husband and I established the first time Caleb left during a meltdown. That occasion resulted with him on the lawn of the neighbor around the corner. She was quite unpleasant in her treatment of Caleb and of us, even when we told her that he is autistic and posed no harm to her. She disagreed and stated that he could pose a threat to her. Caleb was a lean 11-year-old wearing a character t-shirt. She threatened to call the police on us and, in turn, she and I exchanged words.

Luckily, my husband was there to peacefully resolve the situation and remind me that I could be jailed for my actions. His reasoning resonated with me and I backed down, still pissed that she threatened to call the police on us. I could live with her accusing us of being bad parents, but I was greatly troubled by her total lack of empathy and perceptions of a threat from an 11-year-old child. I felt vulnerable, in that even as a mother protecting her child, I knew the woman's threats of police involvement would not work out in my favor.

After the incident, my husband and our close friends developed a plan for managing Caleb's elopements. I would drive north along D Avenue while he would drive north along L Avenue. We would coordinate by phone and search the cross streets. In cases where we needed extra support, we determined that we could call my best friend, who lived a few miles north of our neighborhood. She, along with her teenage son, could provide welcome and trusted faces for Caleb in the event that he wandered.

We put our plan into action and searched the neighborhood at least three times. I called my friend, who sent her husband out to assist in searching for him along busy L Avenue. North to south, south to north we searched and scanned driveways and even stopped into local businesses. We searched to no avail, and an hour later I realized that we needed to call the police, something I dreaded doing for several reasons.

Let me first explain that my husband and I both grew up in low-income tough urban neighborhoods that historically held tenuous relationships with law enforcement. Growing up in our neighborhoods on opposite sides of the city, we both learned that problems were handled by families or by respected individuals in the neighborhood. Calling the cops was the absolute last resort, as they typically were slow to respond or did not respond at all. When the cops did respond, Black residents prepared themselves for situations where asymmetrical power played out with searches, harassment, unproven accusations, or arrests for unrelated matters. Finally, as Black residents of one of the last solidly middle-class neighborhoods in the city, my husband and I faced several situations where police questioned us about our presence in the neighborhood. Husband got hemmed up by the police one evening for simply walking in our driveway and questioned about why he was in the driveway and the neighborhood. In another instance, authorities accused us of stealing the vehicle we reported as smashed and dashed by a drunk driver, despite the fact that I provided proof of ownership. Why would I call regarding an accident if I stole the vehicle? Thus, our experiences as Black people contributed to our unease in calling the police.

I provided a detailed description of Caleb, down to the scar under his eye that he acquired while trying to eat cotton candy while riding a bike. Two hours after he first left home and about 30 minutes after I placed the 911 call, a police vehicle pulled up outside our home. Caleb lumbered out of the back of the police cruiser, hands filled with small plastic animals. Thank God he had the wherewithal to wear a jacket. I was so happy to see him returned in one piece, as I had spent the past 2 hours worried that he had fallen into the hands of an ill-willed pedophile or gang member on D Avenue. My relief, however, was instantly accompanied by familiar pangs of anxiety that arose when I had to deal with the cops. Would they use this occasion to send DHS to our home with the intent of removing my child? Would they interpret Caleb's running away as a criminal act on our part? Will they harass us and accuse us of being bad parents? I recall screaming upstairs to Husband, saying, "He's here! They found him! Grab the bag; we're gonna need it."

In our house, the bag referred to a red and black Vera Bradley paisley patterned bag that contained 2 years' worth of psychological, speech, and behavioral assessments. The bag, in a sense, functioned as my autism passport, in that it held documentation that supported instances of school or public meltdowns. The bag contained proof that we were trying as parents, doing all that we could to access services for Caleb. Thus, the bag provided a protective factor, as my status as a Black mother of a son with autism left me feeling extremely vulnerable to the judgment of providers. In this instance, I hoped the bag provided documentation of my son's condition, our efforts to address his behaviors, and our parental engagement. Call it overreacting but in that instance, I feared my son would be taken away, as many Black mothers had experienced under the judgmental and prejudicial eyes of authorities who deem our approaches to motherhood as pathological.

A sergeant and his trainee approached as I clutched Caleb and the bag. The two then proceeded to relay the story of his 2-mile trek to a public park located across a busy highway. As they told the story, Caleb found his way to the park in a blind rage, calmed down, then approached a nearby ambulance that used the park as a sit-in area while waiting on calls. He introduced himself to the two EMTs, told them that he had left home because he was upset but he had calmed down and was now ready to return. He then told them that he had autism, Tourette's, ADHD, and high anxiety followed by his list of medications. When asked if he was hungry, he replied, "No thanks, I ate before I left home." According to the police, my call went out at about the same time and the EMTs connected with the 911 dispatch to inform them of his whereabouts.

I did get the critical eye from the officers, but once I recognized that I attended Sunday school years ago with the sergeant, the tone changed, and the call ended quickly thereafter. While the police officers shared details of Caleb's excursion, I cried. I was proud of his ability to self-regulate and calm himself. I was extremely proud of his ability to seek out assistance from the EMTs, and especially pleased with how he told HIS story, just the way I taught him with the intention of keeping him safe. He utilized the skills I taught him. I am Caleb's mom and I have to keep him safe.

∼

Across this chapter, Black autism mothers describe similar concerns regarding raising sons at the intersection of race, class, gender, and autism. BAMs engaged in motherwork to ensure their sons' safety, wholeness, and identities. Study participants drew upon protective motherwork strategies such as "the talk" and politicized advocacy to empower their sons. Participants were emboldened by an awareness of how Black mothers are stereotypically maligned, criminalized, and pathologized in American society (Richie, 1999). With these historical and contemporary factors in mind, Black autism mothers in this study were extremely cognizant of the precarious relationship between Black males in American society and law enforcement and shared their fears of police brutality involving their sons (Dottolo & Stewart, 2008; Dow, 2016; Wilson et al., 2004). As Rogers (2015) posits, BAMs' parenting practices are uniquely influenced by an awareness of racial violence targeting Black men, unjust law enforcement interactions, and concerns regarding the perception of autism-related behaviors, combined with race and gender. BAMs centered their maternal practices on keeping their sons safe, as they are profoundly aware that racism is costing lives.

Across study participants, BAMs' love for their sons is highly palpable, almost crushing when considering their fears of how to keep them safe. Michelle reflected upon the vulnerability of Black mothers who must fight to maintain their sons' safety while balancing mothering with additional life stressors. She stated, "There's a vulnerability Black mothers feel whether [our children] have a disability [or not]; the world doesn't treat our children with care. Our children don't walk through the world protected." As such, BAMs describe efforts to keep their sons safe, which speaks to larger concerns about societal misperceptions about Black males' lack of innocence. BAMs counter societal misunderstandings by maintaining exacting standards for their sons, despite autism, as they realize society does not cut Black men slack. BAMs then describe worries of how autism-related behaviors are perceived in public, particularly by law enforcement, and how they subsequently approached the proverbial "talk" that occurs within Black families to prepare sons for police interactions. The chapter will highlight a case involving one participant whose son was racially profiled and physically attacked by a White man.

Protecting the Innocence of Black Boys

Research on Black boyhood illuminates how the lines between Black childhood and adulthood are often blurred, with the adultification and criminalization of Black boys. For Black boys, traditional markers of American childhood are diminished across systems, as Black males experience hypersurveillance (Heitzeg, 2016). Dumas and Nelson (2016), for example, argue that childhood is contextualized in social, political, economic, and cultural milieus, in ways that serve to criminalize Black boys while handling them with a presumed lack of innocence (Dancy, 2014; Goff et al., 2014; Heitzeg, 2016). As evidenced by high adult sentencing rates of adolescents, Black boys in the United States are perceived as adults deserving harsh punishments meted from school disciplinary infractions and the criminal justice system, with little room for rehabilitation or attempts to reframe them as children (Alexander, 2010; Dumas & Nelson, 2016; Heitzeg, 2016). Participating mothers discussed how they were innately aware of how Black boys, including their sons, are perceived as societal threats in schools, the criminal justice system, and society writ large. Furthermore, Heitzeg (2016) argues that race and disability coalesce in negative outcomes for Black boys with criminal justice systems treating them as adults with exacting sentences.

BAMs understood the intricate intersection of race, class, gender, and autism on their sons while also realizing how the intersection positioned both mother and son as vulnerable to punitive measures from schools and law enforcement (Marchand et al., 2019). Mothering at the intersection of being Black, female, and having autistic sons caused BAMs to approach the autism community with caution, as they believed, despite autism, they were still engaging with Whites who lacked an understanding of race. Specifically, BAMs found the representation of autism as a White male condition troublesome, speaking most notably about how images of autism contribute to the public perception that it is exclusively a condition impacting White children and families. BAMs believed that limited representations of autism invisibilized Black children with autism and their families. Lisa, for example, expressed concern that autism is presented as an exclusively White condition, saying, "I think that the face of autism, nationally and locally, is always a little White boy. And I think that, again, people don't often see our kids as vulnerable or deserving of help or compassion, the way other kids are." The framing of autism as a White condition, she believed, subsequently impacts how Black children with autism are perceived and treated across society. The lack of understanding, in her estimation, contributes to BAMs' heightened fears for sons. According to Lisa, mothering at the intersection of race, class, gender, and autism amounts to having "a thousand worries." She further elaborated:

> It's just that danger factor, especially with a boy, it's just that danger factor of, is someone going to harm your child because they don't understand, and they don't have to understand? Because our kids don't have to be understood. Our kids, again, are not deserving of understanding or anything like that. So, I think being a Black mom of an autistic kid, it's just that other element of danger. We're very lucky, being solidly middle class with degrees and jobs, and able to give our kids, able to negotiate the system to get our . . . I know I'm smart enough to know I need a new service coordinator to do some things for me, and how to make a call and how to advocate for my child.

BAMs, unlike mothers of White boys with autism, have the additional safety concern of race, something that cannot be easily addressed by safety strategies such as GPS devices or additional locks to prevent elopement. While these strategies are important, the intersection of race, class, gender, and autism forces BAMs to constantly consider how their sons are not granted the benefit of innocence, thus intensifying safety concerns and keeping them on edge.

Moreover, BAMs were keenly aware of how Black children, particularly Black boys, are adultified by society, meaning they are not given the benefit of innocence associated with childhood, but instead, cast in adult roles (Dancy, 2014; Dumas & Nelson, 2016; Goff et al., 2014; Heitzeg, 2016).

Thus, the behaviors of Black boys are judged through adult lenses, with little room for understanding developmental stages and offering support to assist youth through those stages. Ladson-Billings (2011) describes how social perceptions of Black boys' transitions from an emphasis on cuteness to criminalization, stating:

> The paradox of Black boys' experiences in school and society is that mainstream perceptions of them vacillate between making them babies and making them men. When they are somewhere between the ages of three and six years they are acknowledged as cute but rarely as intellectually capable. This notion of little Black boys as cute does not last long. Before long they are moved to a category that resembles criminals. The fear and control previously referenced appears to be activated and the once "cute" boys become problematic "men." (p. 11)

BAMs noted that while their sons are young and cute, they are not perceived as threats, but instead, as Thelma noted, ". . . when he's small and drooling over himself, he's cute. He's not a threat."

BAMs reflected upon the freedoms associated with innocence and contrasted the adultification of Black boys with the perceived innocence of White boys who grow into adulthood unimpeded by hypersurveillance and negative societal expectations. Michelle elaborated on how such freedoms can function as a spirit killer and an added weight on Black boys. She said, "White children are allowed to be innocent and allowed to be children. There's a freedom that's given to their behaviors that isn't demonized. That doesn't happen for Black children as Black boys are cast as thuggish and threatening. I've witnessed other children have an acceptance or an innocence, an assumed innocence, a freedom to just be, that ours don't. Ours get an expectation, a "What are you doing"? Our children get scrutiny that doesn't happen to others." Dumas and Nelson (2016) mirror Michelle's concerns regarding societal injunctions on Black children seemingly allowed to be children: "Black boys possess their own agential subjectivity and impact the world even as they remain vulnerable to the material effects of racism and the hegemonic notion that their lives as children only matter because of who others want them to be (or fear they may become) in adulthood. Thus, to assert that Black boyhood is unimagined and unimaginable is to lament that we have created a world in which Black boys cannot *be*" (p. 28). As Black boys age and develop, societal views shift from innocence to perceived guilt, menace, and aggression (Dow, 2016). According to the researchers, American society treats Black boyhood as inconceivable and incomprehensible, due to ascribed fears of the Black males they will become in the future (Dancy, 2014; Goff et al., 2014).

Black male stereotypes are transcribed and superimposed upon Black boys, limiting their ability to see themselves or be seen as children. Michelle further fleshed out this point by detailing how prejudice towards Black boys can play out around the special education table. In this instance, Michelle recalled how a White woman at the table described Sam as violent. This accusation enraged Michelle who recalls immediately rejecting the label because the White woman, in a position of authority, invoked a powerful term, which has life-altering outcomes, further demonstrating Dumas and Nelson's (2016) point of "hegemonic notions" impacting life outcomes of Black boys (p. 28). Michelle explained, the use of the term "violent" has long-term consequences for Sam. She said, "I remember correcting them. I told them his behavior is not violent. He is physical and he's big for his age, so if he's having a tantrum and he's kicking or he's jumping or he's throwing his body and you have an aide who is a smaller woman in stature, and she happens to get in the crossfire, that is an example of his autism, but he was not intentionally violent." Michelle believes that her explanation of Sam's behavior spared him being labeled as violent, as she made them remove any description of his behavior as violent from his IEP. Michelle believed the incident also demonstrated that as Black males age, schools lower expectations for positive learning outcomes, withdraw positive attention, and view Black males exclusively through a negative, adultified behavioral lens. She added: "Low expectations. If people have low expectations for our children, as a Black mom, I had that in my mind that I don't just have a child with a disability. I have a Black male who the world already may think that he's coming to the table with less. So, right away, I want to show them what he's coming to the table with." BAMs mothered with an awareness of how Black boys are hypersurveilled in ways that project adulthood on them, while also imposing implicit restrictions upon life outcomes.

Mothering with an Awareness of Police Brutality

Law enforcement safeguarding and inscribing racial codes reaches as far back to the era of enslavement, with images of police brutality toward unarmed Black males ingrained on the American racial consciousness (Alexander, 2010; Whitaker & Snell, 2016). Eric Garner, killed in a police chokehold while mouthing the words "I can't breathe," has become a rallying cry for those seeking to end police brutality and killings of unarmed Black people (Rogers, 2015). The summer of 2020 was also marked by global Black Lives Matter protests in response to the killing of George Floyd by Minneapolis police. And media images of Black mothers mourning, leading curbside vigils, wearing memorial t-shirts, and launching a crescendo of balloons to the sky in the hopes of reaching sons lost to gun violence have become familiar reminders of the perils on young Black lives (Manoucheka, 2018). Rogers (2015) further explains Black mothers' fears as legitimized by historical and contemporary contexts of police brutality and states:

> The traditional framing of police brutality offers little recourse for addressing the harm faced by mothers in the current and historical climate of police brutality, intimidation, and surveillance. This framing requires further examination of the ways mothers of Black men navigate their personal and familial relationship with the police, how they combat negative public perceptions ascribed to Black men and youth, and how they negotiate the safety of their families. The socioeconomic status and racial compositions of the communities where these mothers reside, and whether or not they live in "urban" neighborhoods, will further differentiate their parenting experiences. (p. 211)

BAMs' fears are not unfounded, as several high-profile shootings of Black males with autism have occurred over the past few years. In 2017 for example, Chicago teen Ricardo Hayes was shot and wounded by an off-duty police officer, who initially reported that Hayes approached him in a menacing manner. Watchdog groups and police whistleblowers later revealed the officer's original account of the incident was false and that Hayes did not pose a threat to the officer, who shot the teen through the window of his SUV (Smith, 2020).

Based upon their own experiences and that of Black male family members, including their husbands, participating BAMs were keenly aware of the dangers Black men face as they maneuver through society. Their consciousness was also raised by historical incidents, such as the murder of Emmett Till, and contemporary media coverage of unarmed Black males racially profiled and killed by law enforcement. The cumulative effect was a desire to protect their sons from hegemonic forces of oppression at the hands of law enforcement and other systems. BAMs framed their perspectives on racial profiling of Black males through the eyes of Black males in their lives. As such, given the proximity of racial profiling to their sons, participating mothers worried about the future impact of racism upon their sons. And, as described previously, they sought ways to prepare their sons for racial encounters with the understanding that such incidents are a given in our society. Faith, for example, shared how she listened intently to her husband's stories of having to "dial back," meaning, theoretically reduce his presence to counter racial microaggressions in the workplace. She stated,

> My husband talks about how he's had to sort of almost dial himself down a little bit while he's interacting with work people, because he doesn't want them to think he's being aggressive just when he's being himself. And I feel that would also be a struggle for my son as he got older, when he's just being himself, starting to get into the workforce, or going to school, and him also having autism, because of the kind of challenges it poses, with being able to understand the nuances between other people. And his ability to recognize nonverbal cues. I worry about him being able to pick up on those things, and then others misperceiving him as being either defiant or aggressive.

Faith's fears were further exacerbated by her husband's physical stature, as she described Fat Daddy's size, "He's more than half of my husband's height already, and he's only 7. He is going to definitely be well over 6 ft. My husband is 6 ft. 2 in. He's got the same sort of muscular stature and build as him."

Faith's fears emanated from her husband's experiences navigating the world as a large Black man. She further explained that as Fat Daddy's mother, it was her responsibility to prepare him for how Black men are perceived in American society (Whitaker & Snell, 2016). She added,

> I have to work pretty hard in order to prepare my son to be safe out in the world when I'm not with him. I think about some of the students that I support, and hearing how the teachers describe them, and some of the words that they use are just horrible. And it comes from a place of ignorance, but

thinking about how they are perceived, just because they are Black males with behavioral challenges, knowing that my son sometimes can be defiant, because if he makes it up in his mind that something should be a certain way, he has a hard time understanding that it doesn't always have to be that way, or that even though you might want it to be this way, it's going to have to go according to this person's plan today. And I think about, what happens when my son is in a situation in the community like that, and he's thinking something should be a certain way, and somebody is telling him no, or that it has to go this way, and he's not getting with their program? What's going to happen then?

Sadly, her narrative provides yet another example of how the weight of preparation for intersections of race, class, gender, and autism rests upon Black mothers, as society still racially profiles Black males, even as boys.

"He looks normal," was a shared refrain across all participants, which emerged when participants discussed fears regarding racial profiling. BAMs described their sons' appearances as "normal" to emphasize that society can be unkind when dealing with Black males. They realized their sons' looks would not reveal autism-related challenges of missing social cues, minimal verbal communication, echolalia, or behavioral meltdowns. Across participating mothers of younger sons, BAMs worried that their sons' behaviors would manifest in the future, particularly in terms of racial profiling. Mothers of younger sons, too, continued the refrain of "he looks normal," recognizing that society will not always exercise kindness and patience with their sons' behaviors. They too realized that Black boys grow into Black men who are racially profiled by society.

Donelle disliked the "normal" descriptor but realized that the appearance of "normalcy" and Bear's verbal communication skills add to the semblance that he has the ability to understand law enforcement commands. She stated, "He looks normal. I hate that phrase. But the same person that can discuss politics, conversely, still looks at the Power Rangers. And the political discussion is done with discernment." Her worries were further exacerbated by his small stature, as she elaborated that "he is small and cannot defend himself." Donelle held high standards for her son and credited him with having good sense, or the ability to understand her words regarding safety. She approached that talk as she did with her other son, in a nonformal way, using everyday examples.

She emphasized that "Black men get stopped by the cops." Thus, Donelle realized that the diagnosis of autism does not grant a reprieve to racial profiling that places Black males in precarious situations.

This section highlighted the efforts of BAMs to mitigate and prepare their autistic sons for oppression occurring at the intersection of race, class, gender, and autism. Participating mothers realized that they could, realistically, only control for safety within their homes, as their sons would inevitably confront societal racial microaggressions and injustice (Dumas & Nelson, 2016; Whitaker & Snell, 2016).

Mothering for Safety with "the Talk"

Within Black communities, "the talk" functions as the vehicle for racial socialization, a proverbial rite of passage, with Black parents teaching their children racial rules of engagement (DiAquoi, 2017; Whitaker & Snell, 2016). The "talk," which is typically historically situated with parents drawing upon the lessons of previous generations' racial encounters, teaches children how to interact with law enforcement, compete in the marketplace, dress, speak, and develop awareness of racial dangers (DiAquoi, 2017). The talk is intended to keep Black children safe from racial harm by teaching them to navigate situations and diminish or avoid racialized interactions with more powerful Whites. Safety in this sense includes emotional, psychological, and physical (DiAquoi, 2017). In this sense, the talk is predicated upon the presumption of *when* a racial infraction occurs versus *if* a racial infraction could ever occur. It is also premised on Black parents' ability to verbally communicate the ways in which larger educational, criminal justice, and political systems were fundamentally not intended to work toward the benefit of Black people (Barnes, 2016; Heitzeg, 2016; Whitaker & Snell, 2016).

Black mothers of autistic sons, in delivering the talk, must account for their sons' ability to comprehend the context of race in America. BAMs and their families must also discern how best to convey behavioral awareness to sons who struggle with interpreting social cues and appropriate reciprocal communication. The talk occurs in Black families regardless of class and social standing as demonstrated by Hollywood actress Holly Robinson Peete and her husband, retired NFL quarterback Rodney Peete. The Peetes filmed a popular reality television show centered on family.

The show featured a dedicated storyline focused on their son RJ's coming of age as a young man on the autism spectrum. The family supports RJ as he learns to drive and strives for independence. In one episode, Holly and Rodney sit RJ down at the family table, a safe comfortable space, and review with him step-by-step police commands, with a demonstration of how to raise his hands, show his identification, and respond to police commands (DiAquoi, 2017). When asked what he would do if he got scared during a police stop, RJ responded, "I would call my mommy," to which Holly patiently replied, "Umm no, because then you would have to reach into your pocket to get your phone." The Peetes use clear, step-by-step directives as they guide RJ through a series of different scenarios. The couple genuinely feared for RJ's safety and did not believe their celebrity would buffer him from police brutality.

Similarly, BAMs tailored the talk to their sons' personalities, social skills, and communication abilities. Participating mothers of older sons, like the Peetes, faced a conundrum of wanting to honor and develop their sons' independence, while placing freedoms within a racialized context. BAMs want their sons to have some semblance of independence, particularly in mothers of sons with high-functioning autism, as the young men are cognizant of the markers of adolescence and adulthood. BAMs' sons, like RJ, desire freedoms such as walking home from school or jobs. The Black parenting strategy of the talk became increasingly germane to helping sons understand that freedoms for Black men in this country come with risks to their safety and well-being.

The talk within Indigo's household centered on the safety that home provides, a place offering protection from the harm of the outside world. Indigo shared how her family resides in an all-White suburban neighborhood. She made a point of making sure that Poobie, 17, knows all the neighbors to ensure that the neighbors are cognizant of Poobie's autism. Indigo does not take for granted that strangers drive through her neighborhood: strangers who could potentially misinterpret Poobie's behaviors or report him to authorities as a threat. Her fears were exacerbated by the fact that Poobie now walks home alone from school, a proud achievement for him. Indigo, like many Black mothers, balanced out Poobie's burgeoning independence with concerns for his safety. Thus, she associated the talk with Poobie's house key, teaching him that no matter what happens outside their doors, the house provides safety and sanctuary. She described her vigilance (Spano et al., 2011) by sharing,

> That key is huge. I really believe that that obsession of ours is because he's a young Black boy. [I tell him], "You got to have the ability to get in the sanctuary of your house. That is not an option for you," particularly again, people are like, "Well, he's not growing up in the hood, what you worried about"? [I'm] worried about White folk more than Black people. He's a tall young Black man. Now, the people in my immediate neighborhood know who he is, but you never know who's driving through those streets.

Indigo's "obsession" with the house key also demonstrates a realization of the limitations of her control, as she can control safety issues within her home, but she also recognized that she could not control for racial profiling immediately outside the home.

Lisa did not take for granted that her sons would encounter police in her suburban neighborhood. For example, she shared how her older son was racially profiled by police under suspicion of being a burglar. While walking home from school, the teen was thrown on a police car, cuffed, and questioned. Police then took her underage son to the scene of the crime for identification by the victims, who fortunately did not identify him as the suspect. Her son was then placed back in the police car and dropped off at her home. She was never contacted by authorities to explain their actions. She shared this story as a contrast to reflect on how John would have fared in the same situation:

> At least he knew enough to comply, which I don't think he should have, but for his own safety, he complied. He showed them his ID. He got in the car with them, went to this man's house, because I think he knew, "Well I didn't do anything wrong." Then afterward the police were like, "Oh, you know, our bad. Can we, can we drop you off somewhere?" So, he's like, "Yeah, drop me off at home." So police drop him off, like no harm no foul. I'm livid, I'm pissed off, I'm mad. My oldest is sort of like, "Oh well. It's over."

While her oldest son was able to dismiss the incident and was released, physically unscathed, the occurrence left a lasting imprint upon Lisa, who realized that John would have encountered difficulties if placed in the same situation. The ending could have been far worse if John were accosted and accused of a crime. Lisa's oldest son took the talk to heart, complying with commands and showing his ID. In the case of John, however, Lisa worries about his ability to comply, especially given his minimal verbal communication and social skills. She explained,

> I worry about John, because of course he's not very verbal, and he might have a sudden movement with the arm twitching. He can't comply with, "Freeze" or "Stop." He might take off and run if he were in that kind of situation. We've heard stories of how police have shot disabled people, developmentally disabled people, or mentally ill people, and so that is my fear, is that if he were sort of somehow out there in the community without someone with him to sort of translate or be with him . . . the police mistake his actions for aggressive and threatening, and shoot him or harm him or something, or arrest him or something like that? Because John does not understand these things, of course, can't comply. So, then the police could theoretically harm my child and get away with it.

Lisa responded to her fears in a manner similar to Indigo, establishing a sphere of safety with stringent safety practices where family can control what happens to John (Spano et al., 2011). Society at large represented a place where John was susceptible to racial profiling, in a manner similar to his brother. Lisa and Indigo's experiences highlight that despite BAMs' efforts to protect their sons by controlling their immediate settings, BAMs recognized that they could not control for societal racial bias and subsequent racial profiling. The realization, however, did not stop their protective efforts (Whitaker & Snell, 2016).

Fueled by the underlying realization that their sons' behaviors will be viewed through a racialized lens, some BAMs described efforts to address and improve their sons' behaviors. For Karla, mothering two sons with autism proved challenging, especially when dealing with autism-related behaviors. Her youngest, 6-year-old Mikey, as a result of minimal verbal communications, was physically aggressive with peers, even bloodying a child's nose. In another instance, Mikey stomped on a teacher's toe out of frustration, subsequently breaking the woman's toe. Karla worried about the long-term impact of Mikey's behaviors, specifically, whether the behaviors would lead to police interactions. She said,

> My husband and I fear their safety, especially for Mikey because he is sometimes aggressive or is not able to articulate and

communicate to say what he needs or wants . . . he'll get upset and frustrated and *people can't see their disabilities* [emphasis added]. They are perceived as being an angry Black male. Right now, in this country, that could get you hurt or killed, just by expressing your frustration, people perceive you as being hostile or aggressive when you're just expressing your frustrations.

Here again, the intersection of race, class, gender, physical stature, and autism intersect, as Karla expressed a concern that Black boys cannot simply be boys with the presumption of innocence (Dumas & Nelson, 2016; Heitzeg, 2016). Given the hypersurveillance of Black boys, visible disabilities do not insulate Black males on the autism spectrum from racially motivated harm.

Karla found a mental health therapist for Mikey and he receives in-home behavioral therapy. She believes the therapy, coupled with medicine, are helping him to better handle his frustration. And despite the young ages of 6-year-old Mikey and 11-year-old Andrew, Karla has attempted to have the talk with them based upon the history of race in the US. She explained, "My husband and I are harder on the boys and may at times have higher expectations for [them] than maybe they can meet at times, because we fear their safety with police. We hear things that are happening such as race relations, which have always been present in this country but are really even more prevalent right now."

Karla further explained that in attempting to have the talk with her boys, Andrew is better equipped to understand due to his age, and the fact that his in-school history curriculum has touched upon racism. She elaborated, however, that while he is better equipped to understand, she still does not believe that he fully comprehends discussions of racism. "I talk to him about how it's still present, how he could be perceived in this country, anywhere in the world, as a young Black male. I don't think he really understands. He feels bad about it, when we talk about racism and how people are treated, but he doesn't really understand. It's hard." Karla's fears illuminate paradoxes at the intersection of race, class, gender, and autism with social expectations that Black boys understand race, which is further complicated by autism.

Similarly, Thelma shared her experiences dealing with two sons on the autism spectrum with challenging behaviors. Thelma recognized that interpretations of Black boys' behaviors as violent and perceptions of their physical appearances contribute to their imperiled status. She noted how her fears are now punctuated given 14-year-old Elijah's stature, saying, "He's now over 6 feet tall, 14 years old, and has hormones." While Elijah is quiet and introspective, Thelma worries constantly about how 7-year-old Solomon, who is also diagnosed with Tourette's syndrome, will fare in society as a Black male, based upon his behaviors. For example, Solomon often uses curse words to verbally express his frustration with school preparation and attendance. Thelma shared how it was not unusual for him to say, "Shut up bitch," and throw things at her each morning as she prepared him for school. She elaborated that with prayer and behavioral and speech therapy, Solomon's behaviors and language have greatly improved, and he is now better able to express his frustrations, thereby decreasing meltdowns. She reflected on the shift in his behaviors and language, saying, "God is so amazing and makes us so brilliantly that we have so many different ways to get our points across." Thelma does, however, continue to worry about the safety of her sons.

Participants realized that the talk was ongoing and situational, meaning they reinforced the message of the larger talk with racial messaging situated in the context of social settings. Thus, the talk was not necessarily a one-and-done conversation but was frequently revisited as BAMs prepared sons for different social settings. Ginger referred to situational talks as "mini-orientations" that occur prior to entering public settings. Mini-orientations prepared her adult sons, Cat Man and Music Man, for social interactions. She elaborated: "I tell him we have to be careful. We have the orientation in the car. When we pull up to the restaurant, before we go to church. Mini-orientations prepare them for how we're going to conduct ourselves and what we're going to say." Ginger was especially worried about Cat Man's social interactions, as he does not fully understand social cues and personal space. She expressed that "socially, [they] are still working on Cat Man because he feels like everyone is a friend."

Ginger's concerns about Cat Man's behaviors also raise an important point about BAMs' unique positionality among mothers of sons with autism. BAMs, like many mothers of Black sons, strategized racial safety with the talk. In addition to addressing their sons' social, communicative, and physical constraints associated with autism, BAMs had the added burden of translating the talk into behavioral modifications to protect their sons from racial profiling and other forms of racial violence. Ginger's concerns were heightened in the wake of Black Lives Matter protests, when a family friend decided he could no longer take Cat Man on social outings. As conveyed by Ginger, the friend believed,

> In the event that an emergency occurred, Cat Man will walk up to the officer like, "Hello officer, I think you're doing a marvelous job." *There was no filter we could create to keep him safe* [emphasis added]. [Our friend] was concerned that if something happened, he wouldn't be able to explain Cat Man's behaviors, the way they've been so trigger happy here lately. We've raised our children to honor and respect authority. You don't have to be afraid because you're not doing wrong but our friend felt he wouldn't have control over his behaviors because he's so friendly. He's tall and handsome. People don't know that there are these deficits he's working through. They just see a tall Black man coming up to them.

Ironically, she realized that Cat Man's kind and friendly nature could ultimately place him in danger given societal perceptions of his race, class, gender, physical stature, and autism, an intersection shaped by unreasonable and inequitable social expectations. The intersection ladened BAMs with inscribing race-safe behaviors on sons who struggle to even recognize racial constraints imposed on Black men while simultaneously acknowledging that there are no "filters" to keep her son safe. Subsequently, the family friend and Ginger agreed that ending the outings was in Cat Man's best interests.

It should be noted that BAMs did not fault their sons for autism-related behaviors, as they sought to develop and honor their respective personalities. Racially underscored behavioral modifications were, however, an attempt to buffer sons from a pervasive lack of society's understanding at the intersection of race, class, gender, and autism. BAMs recognized that they could not control for societal responses and interpretations of their sons' behaviors but they could enact elements of the talk (Dumas & Nelson, 2016). In the case of Cat Man, behavioral modification, in some ways, meant dimming a facet of his personality to shelter him from harm. Sadly, talk and behavioral modifications cannot guarantee safety, freedom, and the ability to live unburdened by the threat of racialized violence. The next section speaks to this point and BAMs' worst fears actualized—a physical attack at the intersection of race, class, gender, and autism.

A True-to-Life Experience at the Intersection of Race, Class, Gender, and Autism

On a crisp October morning, Pappas Charles literally ran directly into the intersection of race, disability, and gender.[1] Candi traveled with Pappas to a midsize city, where he participated in an early morning cross-country meet sponsored by a historically Black fraternity. Pappas loves to run and, as Candi shared, found himself and a community of caring peers through running. His teammates welcomed him and helped him acclimate to the team's social dynamics and expectations. Although he is not a record-breaking runner, long runs provided Pappas much-needed sensory integration. His parents exposed him to a variety of activities, but Pappas immediately took to distance running. Candi usually ran with him, but due to an injury, she was unable to accompany Pappas on the run that morning.

Unfortunately, Pappas became lost, wandered off course, and reportedly approached a car with a White married couple, seeking assistance. According to police reports, the White man, 57, exited his vehicle and confronted Pappas. In one police report, the man said that he feared Pappas was going to mug his wife, despite the fact that the couple sat in their car. The man later shared with law enforcement that his car was recently broken into by "youths" and that incident lingered in his mind. He rationalized his violent actions toward Pappas based on the break-in and told police the incident caused him to be apprehensive of Pappas. Despite protestations of his fears, the man emerged from his car and stood directly in Pappas's face. Subsequently, the man stated that he was unaware of Pappas's autism and believed the young man was on drugs due to his echolalia, minimal verbal communication, and autism-related body movements, which he interpreted as "strange." He then proceeded to push Pappas to the ground and reared back to punch him until stopped by two concerned bystanders, who wrote down the man's license plate information. The man was described by the bystanders as having a large frame, heavyset, and tall.

---

1. The details of this incident that did not come from Candi were widely reported in the city's local press and even drew national attention. (To keep Pappas's identity confidential, I did not specify the city or the newspaper that much of the information came from.)

Due to a series of jurisdictional mix-ups, a judge declined to sign an arrest warrant for the man. Frustrated and angered at the lack of justice, Candi reported the incident to her city council member, which led to the story gaining press attention. Several reporters from Candi's hometown traveled to the city to further investigate the incident. Candi's councilwoman reached out via letter to the district attorney, demanding an explanation as to why the man had not been arrested. Additionally, the story was then picked up by the national media because it served as yet another instance of a Black male being profiled and violated with no resulting action on the part of law enforcement. Candi vehemently pressed for justice, believing that if the case involved a Black man who pushed a White boy, the outcome would be quite different. With increased attention and bad press, law enforcement, along with the district attorney, revisited the assault. Given that the incident occurred within the city limits and the man resided in a neighboring suburban town, confusion between police agencies resulted in an insufficient report that thereby prevented the presiding judge from moving forward with charges. The original report by city officers contained scant details and omitted details that county sheriff's deputies later included in their reporting, which then allowed for charges to be pressed against Pappas's assailant.

In the days following the incident, several notable events occurred. First, Pappas turned in his cross-country uniform; he did not want to run anymore. Candi rallied to encourage him and worked to help Pappas regain a sense of safety and confidence, as understandably, the situation was traumatic. Never one to rest on her laurels, Candi and other members of Pappas's family organized an autism run in his community to increase autism awareness. As the case gained media attention, the police force in the city where the incident occurred made attempts to repair damages to Pappas and their reputation due to the botched incident reporting. Officers traveled to Pappas's home to get a statement from Candi endeavoring to produce a more accurate report that could then lead to charges against the assailant. After learning that Candi wanted Pappas to continue running, the police force organized a run with police academy recruits. Pappas ran at the front of the pack. Finally, Candi organized a spin class where community members could meet, interact, and exercise with Pappas.

During the maelstrom, Candi received letters of support that poured in from across the region, state, and country. Although I did not know Candi at that time, I wrote the district attorney in the city to speak out about the lack of justice. I also sent the letter to Candi along with a letter of support for her, as I wanted her to know she was not alone. Unfortunately, the incident also garnered some negative attention with a variety of naysayers questioning why Pappas ran the race alone. What the naysayers did not realize is that Candi prepared Pappas for the race by walking the course with him prior to the start of the race. She typically ran races with him but could not run that particular day due to a knee injury. The incident, according to Candi, was not about Pappas being unaccompanied on a run, but was about implicit racial bias. The man pleaded guilty to endangering the welfare of a child, a misdemeanor, and second-degree harassment. He was sentenced to 80 hours of community service, 3 years of probation, and a 5-year no-contact order during which he is prohibited from contacting Pappas and the Charles family. At the sentencing, the man shared that he was unaware of Pappas's autism and read a prepared statement expressing his remorse. He did not make mention of Pappas's race and gender as a determining factor for his violent actions.

Throughout the ordeal, Candi pressed for justice by bringing the story to the attention of the media, keeping the story in the spotlight, and sustaining her insistence upon justice. Even though the US criminal justice system functions with hegemonic interests in mind, Candi wanted Pappas's humanity recognized and the White assailant brought to justice. Shortly after the verdict, Candi stood before the local media cameras, looking somewhat relieved that justice had been served, and summarized the entire episode:

> I appreciated what the judge had to say, as far as when he saw my son, his biases were there, and that's why he did what he did to him. I did appreciate his letter, it was just a little too late. I'm glad that this chapter is closed. I have to continue to deal with raising my son. And yes, he's back to running . . . his running helps his school and helped him get through his daily life. It's still hard. There are people I have to pay to run with him. There are programs that I have to put him in to run with him that are more special. Staff members at school that are being paid extra to run with him. So, it's now like, "Oh he's back to running." It's a lot of work. More work than it was on October 13th [the day before the incident]. But this chapter is closed.

Candi's words highlight what the public at large failed to understand: Pappas does not run to gain accolades or prizes. Instead, some commenters attempted to blame Candi for Pappas running alone, illuminating what Richie (1999) characterizes as a pathologizing of Black mothers. Running, instead, served the purpose of regulating his body, providing a means to focus and socialize with peers. Thus, running was essential to his very being, in a social, emotional, physical, and vestibular sense. These things could have easily been lost that day at the hands of an aggressive, hate-filled White man.

When we sat down and discussed the incident, Candi reflected on how angry she was that Pappas had been violated, an innocent Black child assaulted by a cowardly racist. She struggled with how to explain the situation to him, but settled upon the following: "I always reinforce positive into him. 'You know why that man did that? Because you have this color skin, and he has that color skin. He thinks everybody with this color skin is bad. This man did this because he didn't like the color of your skin. But that's not true, right? That's not true.' He knows that, and I had to teach him. I said, 'Pappas, there's going to be nice people and there's going to be mean people.'" After the story gained traction in the local, regional, and national media, Pappas received an outpouring of kindness and gifts from people who were outraged by the story. Candi did not take the kindness of others for granted and used it to show Pappas that good people still exist. She described how she sits with Pappas and opens mail, saying, "You know, we read every letter, every gift he opened it himself. And I said, 'Look at how many nice people [there are]. And there's that one person. So just try to remember that. There's going to be nice people, there's going to be mean people. But I hope there's more nice people.'" Candi sent thank-you notes to all who sent letters and packages to Pappas and included a picture of Pappas smiling and holding his cross-country jersey.

In retrospect, Candi reflected on how she prepared him to navigate people's perceptions of him as a young man with autism. When Pappas was 8, Candi sought to understand how he viewed himself and autism in relation to his peers. She said, "He knows that he's special. He knows he's different. I asked him that. I think he was about 8. I said, 'Pappas, do you know that you're different?' And he's like, 'Yes.' So, he knows he's different."

The incident at the cross-country meet, however, deprived her of the opportunity of explaining to Pappas how race, class, gender, and autism intersect to impact how others might treat him. The event left her upset that the opportunity to have the talk with Pappas from a preventative stance, as opposed to in response to a racially charged incident, was taken away, as Pappas encountered the intersection of race, class, gender, autism, and hate in that incident. "I wanted to be the one to pick and choose about racism." Shortly after Pappas was attacked, she redirected her energies to engaging Pappas in the talk, this time using documentaries and movies to illuminate how Whites historically treated Blacks. She commented:

> How can I tell [Pappas] to hate White people? But it's so easy for them to want to hate us, just because. So what we did is even when they were doing slavery in school, and stuff, I had him pulled out the class. And we watched *Eyes on the Prize*. And we watched the new one, the African Voyage. I think it was four parts. We watched the one that Spike Lee did. We would watch stuff and then I would explain to him. Then I would come up with ways. I definitely had to teach him what my mother taught me. "You treat people how they treat you, no matter what color they are." She said, "There's going to be Black people you not going to like, and there's going to be Asian people you not going to like, but you just treat people the way they treat you."

Thus, Candi approached "the talk" using media references, questions, and the reminder to treat people as you expect to be treated.

The incident demonstrates, again, how young Black men, by virtue of race and gender, do not receive the benefit of innocence; thereby illuminating how the fears of BAMs can easily become a reality. DiAngelo (2018), for example, argues that Whites perceive Blacks as inclined to commit crimes against them, thus, engendering deep-rooted fears justified by racist beliefs. Speaking from the perspective of White privilege, DiAngelo states, "Deeply held white associations of black people with crime distort reality and the actual direction of danger that has historically existed between whites and blacks. The vast history of extensive and brutal explicit violence perpetrated by whites and their ideological rationalizations are all trivialized white claims of racial innocence. The power we now wield and have wielded for centuries is thus obscured" (p. 186). In other words, there is a belief that young Black men, who are predisposed to commit crime, deserve retribution for simply being Black and male. Or, in the case of Pappas, Black, male, and autistic. The man acted out his racialized fears of young Black men as he exacted violence on Pappas, reifying his White superiority and the perceived inhumanity of young Black men (DiAngelo, 2018). The delayed response of the justice system, along with the poor reporting of law enforcement also speaks to the ways in which systems function with hegemonic interests at the intersection of race, class, gender, and autism.

Chapter Summary

Black autism mothers described how mothering at this intersection is an exponential political act with BAMs decidedly approaching mothering strategies to counter negative social expectations and perceptions of their sons, while strategizing on how to keep their sons protected. Participants recognized that Black boys are not afforded childhoods but instead are adultified and subjected to hypersurveillance (Dancy, 2014). BAMs amended the talk, a form of racial preparation, to their sons' social skills, communication abilities, personalities, and comprehension level. Participants mitigated the balance between personal development with safety concerns, which led mothers to extend the talk to directed behavioral modifications. Despite such efforts, one participant shared the story of her son's tragic encounter shaped by negative perceptions of Black males. BAMs also realized that their sons' autism further complicates how Black males are treated in this society. Thus, Black autism mothers must also mitigate the intersection of race, class, gender, and autism.

Chapter 5

Education at the Intersection of Race, Class, Gender, and Autism

Daycare. Pre-K early intervention gave Caleb his voice. Taught him the fundamentals. Taught me a new autism vocabulary. He loves school.

K–2. Let's repeat kindergarten because socially he is not quite ready for first grade. Caleb can do the work but struggles socially. He absolutely must have an aide to help him transition and maintain focus across the day. I help with homework. I accompany the class on field trips. I attend every school event. I show up during the day. I maintain a regular presence at the school. Miss Wilson, an old friend of my mother, is Caleb's aide. Thank you for letting me know the teachers spoke despairingly of me. The focus should be upon Caleb. Meltdowns started. The meds will help him focus and remain calm. Occupational therapy reintroduces a sensory diet—weighted vest, brushing, gently pulling finger joints, and yoga ball rolls. Isn't there an autism classroom at the elementary school? Yes, but it is self-contained. Where will he attend school next? I reach out to my social network and he lands a coveted spot at the top elementary school in the district. White parents covet placements in the school. He deserves to be here as much as anyone else. I will not be guilted for my advocacy.

Grades 3–6, or was it fifth grade? This is where the blur really started. Gen ed classroom with push-in supports doesn't seem to be enough. Speech continues to focus on strengthening oral musculature. Straws help. Miss Adrienne develops a routine of self-monitoring drooling. "Keep a napkin with you at all times Caleb." Adjustments to the sensory diet needed. He does pretty well academically. Marked uptick and intensity of behaviors. Med adjustments are necessary to help him get through the day. Anxiety is high. Perseverative behaviors and endless echoes of "I'm sorry, I'm sorry" interrupt his day and shut down teaching. Transitions are hard even with Miss Adrienne's and Miss Melissa's assistance. Pull-out specialist time increases. Hospitalization.

Advocate for that private school placement for students with learning disabilities. Oh yes, we work with students on the spectrum. The district will cover tuition expenses and transportation is provided. Sense of relief. He can stay here for high school. Gorgeous building, but I notice students and parents do not look like us. Private school for half of sixth grade. This isn't working. Calls every day. If they can't reach me, they call my mother. Come get him. Keep him out for a few days. No one seems interested in his success. Suspended for a week. Anxiety. OCD-isms. Excoriation. Nail beds bleed. Picking away at himself to ease anxiety. "I'm sorry, I'm sorry" worsens and takes over his growing body like a possession. Meltdowns intensify. Elopements escalate and safety concerns reached a critical point. Hard stop. Second hospitalization. Private school dismisses him. No assistance with subsequent placement.

District tutors and me, the remainder of sixth grade. I cannot get answers to what options are available. At wit's end. He needs to be in school and no one seems to have answers. Social network points me to a therapeutic day treatment program for middle school. The placement is out of district, housed in a suburban district. Damn, yet another fight. Got the placement—therapeutic day treatment in an out-of-district placement for half of seventh grade.

Hard stop with schooling and living arrangements. Transition to group home living and a rural school. Can they provide a quality education? There are only a handful of Black kids out here. Will he be treated well? Staff share assurances that he will be well taken care of and respected. "Caleb, look at the cornfields across the street from the school. You cannot run through the hallways and elope into the cornfields. You cannot join the children of the corn. It will be difficult to locate you and will require a crop duster." He smiled and nodded indicating that he understood. "You're funny Mom."

High school. He transitions into the other district building. The continued dilemma of an academic program or training program. Academic program will position him for college. Community college? Training program? Hmm, maybe I know too much about the history of Black education, so this option doesn't feel right in my spirit. Besides, mechanical work is not an option. The family and house staff are still working on hygiene issues, so food service is out. "Caleb, I know you have anxiety, but you cannot take off your shoes and pick at your feet." "Typhoid Caleb. Mom that's funny."

Caleb can do the work and meet state standards. The academic program is really the only choice. But, students in his autism program typically do not pursue a Regents diploma. We will be sure he gets socioemotional supports in social group with the other boys enrolled in the autism program. We will be sure he gets academic supports. I have heard promises from schools before, especially that dreadful private school. I do not easily trust that school personnel will function in the best interest of my son.

Social group is a favorite—a space where he blossoms. He becomes the mouthpiece for classmates who cannot speak up for themselves. He helps students with physical disabilities. He encourages classmates when they are sad. Caleb experiences exponential socioemotional growth.

Fingers crossed for the state exams. Anxiety is off the chain. He struggles. But he prevails. They kept their promises about respect, and academic and socioemotional supports. I am pleased and grateful.

High school graduation. I knew the day would be emotional. A mascara-free day. Why play around with Kleenex? I brought a hand towel. We rolled into the graduation deep—20 strong and all proud of Caleb. Family from out of state attend. He had a squad of folks cheering him on when he walked across the stage to receive his Regents diploma: the lone Regents graduate among his peer group.

In preparation for this chapter, I reflected upon Caleb's schooling experiences. Unlike the other chapters with well-crafted narratives, I could not think or write fluently about his school experiences. Stream of consciousness fell into my spirit and flowed, as I realized an effortless narrative was not possible because the 16-year journey from daycare, pre-K, elementary, middle, and high school was not seamless, easy, or smooth. It was a disjointed journey strung together by social networking, luck, and prayer. God protects babies and fools, as the expression goes.

Caleb's schooling journey, however, captures the uncertainty that parents of children with autism face, particularly regarding school placements, programs, staffing, and resources. The battles for services are endless, but so are the corresponding skirmishes for respect. But there were some people along the way; teachers, aides, therapists, school psychologists, nurses, and counselors who worked valiantly on Caleb's behalf. I am eternally grateful as their presence made all the difference on that bumpy disjointed schooling journey.

I am weary yet resilient. I am Caleb's mom.

∼

The historical record documents Black mothers' political activism for equitable education and quality schooling choices for Black children. Black mothers who engage in motherwork approach their children's education with an awareness that American schools are sites of social reproduction (Allen & White-Smith, 2018; Wilson Cooper, 2007). The political activism of Black mothers is further undergirded by concerns about educational outcomes, with mothers clearly understanding the high-stakes connection of schooling and access to greater economic and social opportunities. For Black mothers of sons with autism, political activism is heightened by the fight for equitable access to special education services, including school choice, classroom placements, and educational resources (Morgan & Stahmer, 2020; Stanley, 2015). BAMs of school-aged sons in this study unequivocally demonstrated how education at the intersection of race, class, gender, and autism necessitated political action to address asymmetrical power relations between schools and parents.

Research on Black mothers and school partnerships highlights the ways in which schools misinterpret actions and counter Black mothers with adverse actions and authoritative positions, thereby shifting the focus away from the child (Chapman & Bhopal, 2013; Rowley et al., 2010). This section will describe how BAMs strategize to navigate school systems, as they seek appropriate services for their sons. Wilson Cooper (2007) speaks to the specificities of school advocacy by addressing how Black mothers' identities, or perceptions thereof, are inextricably linked to power: "The mothers' valuing of education and their experiences with inequity have caused them to take a defensive position in the educational marketplace. Their narratives reflect a tenet of Black feminist theory that suggests that Black women's positionality usually disadvantages them given their membership in multiple marginalized groups (Black, female and often poor). Thus, in line with the notion of motherwork, the mothers' identity and that of their children matter" (p. 502).

Black mothers, therefore, enter school systems viewed not as equal partners but seen as subordinates, based upon their social identities. As Chapman and Bhopal (2013) argue, Black parents take oppositional stances in school settings in response to presumptions held of them by White educators. For BAMs in this study, oppositional stances were necessary to counter negative perceptions of White educators. In some instances, BAMs learned of teachers and other school staff speaking negatively of them, perceiving BAMs as oppositional, attitudinal, and unable to partner with teachers and school leaders (Wilson Cooper, 2007).

Black Mothers' Involvement with Special Education

Special education adds yet another layer to the complex obstacles Black mothers encounter while navigating school systems. Hyper-referrals of Black children to special education, in particular Black boys, for disciplinary infractions and other subjective measures, is not lost on Black mothers (Allen & White-Smith, 2018; Artiles et al., 2002). Parental involvement in special education, particularly that of Black parents, is further complicated by barriers including failures in effective written communication, English-only communications, inconvenient scheduling of meetings, and disregard for parental input on critical decisions (Kalyanpur et al., 2000). School failures may also be met with resistance from parents frustrated by previous negative interactions, language barriers, and resistance to the diagnosis (Kalyanpur et al., 2000).

Under ideal circumstances, parents of children with autism remain in regular contact with their child's educational team, regularly exchanging in two-way communication to support mutually established learning and behavioral outcomes. Communication between teachers, support staff, and parents also facilitates information exchange leading up to annual Committee on Special Education (CSE) meetings, during which the child's IEP is written. The IEP table, by law, is supposed to include parents, allowing them to share knowledge of their child's strengths and weaknesses, contextualized by a full and authentic picture of their child's out-of-school life (Fish, 2006). Educators should attend these annual meetings ready to engage parents from a strengths-based perspective, sharing special education expertise as complementary points to parents' insights of their child. Other school staff members, including the school psychologist, an administrator, and even the school nurse share observational and evaluation data (Fish, 2009). If the child is over the age of 14, they are involved and allowed to speak during the meeting. Agreements are reached about the child's educational program, as evidenced in intentional classroom or program placements in which the child can thrive.

The annual meeting description provided above is an idealized version of events, devoid of racial, gendered, and classed contexts in which Black women engage in motherwork (Collins, 1994). The idealized description also fails to consider innate power struggles between parents and school staff related to parental knowledge, professional knowledge, and what lies between both forms of knowledge (Kalyanpur et al., 2000). Lopez (2014) argues that teachers specifically function as "gateway providers" (p. 21), meaning they wield power in knowing what services are availed in districts to special education students. Teachers' recommendations, along with that of other staff members, carry considerable weight in determining not only IEP contents but how the IEP will be enacted. Furthermore, annual meetings are often the culmination of parental involvement across the academic year and reflect ongoing parent-teacher interactions. Said otherwise, if parents and school staff have not sustained positive and productive communications across the school year, subsequent formal special education meetings may only serve to exacerbate and calcify such differences. IEP meetings may also fail to yield fitting educational placements and depend heavily upon school district resources, staffing, and a menu of classroom placement options.

From a parental perspective, annual CSE meetings may trigger anxiety, frustration, feelings of disrespect, and marginalization, as Black parents advocate for their children in a contested space. Fish (2006, 2009) notes that it is not unusual for parents to become overwhelmed by the jargon used to describe evaluation results; district/school special education services; the frequency of services; and individualized socioemotional, physical, and learning outcomes. Additionally, although parents are supposed to play a critical role in crafting shared educational goals, parental involvement is further questionable if decisions regarding placements and services are made prior to the annual meeting, in conversations far removed from parents (Cooper & Christie, 2005).

Across this chapter, Black autism mothers describe the perils of navigating special education services for their sons. BAMs provide a detailed picture of the complexities of parental involvement, noting how their presence is not always met with pleasantries, partnership, and positive outcomes (Kalyanpur et al., 2000). BAMs illuminated how race, class, gender, and autism intersect within schooling contexts, as participants described blatant affronts to Black mothers, with some BAMs reporting judgment, scrutiny, and educators' attempts to minimize parental input on key decisions. Conversely, BAMs' narratives provide insights on Black mothers' willingness to partner with schools, highlighting relational elements that earn their trust. BAMs who were successful in building trusting relationships with schools demonstrate how sustained engagements, information sharing, and mutual respect directly benefited their sons' educational outcomes. Participants recognized the importance of BAMs' experiential knowledge and standpoints and sought out ways to share their knowledge of special education and autism with other Black parents. The chapter concludes with an in-depth consideration of power dynamics between BAMs and schools and highlights a case of power gone awry, resulting in a traumatic incident.

BUILDING TRUST WITH BAMS

Participating Black mothers were keenly aware of the historically precarious relationship between Black mothers and school staff and, accordingly, approached schools with suspicion (Lareau & Horvat, 1999). BAMs looked for behaviors and discursive cues demonstrating sincerity and genuine interest in their sons; such indicators opened them to developing trusting relationships. Collaborating with school staff entailed building trusting relationships on nonjudgmental interactions and sustained positive communications (Pearson & Meadan, 2021).

At the start of each school year, Kiara assessed Johnathan's teachers to determine their sincerity and her willingness to trust them. Kiara attended class field trips under the guise of providing extra support for Johnathan during outings, with teachers and Johnathan believing she was there to "hang out with him." To the contrary, Kiara used field trips to assess his teachers, as she believed the outings and school appearances allowed her to see, as she noted, "What kind of teacher are you? What kind of adult are you? Not even what kind of teacher you are. Are you attentive? Are you biased? Do you have classroom favorites?" In doing so, Kiara believed she was acting out advice received years ago from another BAM, who shared, "You are the expert on your child. They're only with him 3 hours, 4 hours, but you raise him, you know him, you live with him. If they say something that's contrary to that, then you need to speak up and never forget that." The field trips allowed her to exercise discernment about Johnathan's teachers and demonstrate her school presence.

BAMs' interactions with teachers also highlights the delicate balance of autism knowledge, specifically, as maternal and school-based autism knowledge are often positioned as being oppositional. The balance of power plays out in school communications, with BAMs expressing frustration and distrust. BAMs perceived daily negative communications from teachers as an unnecessary annoyance and resulted in them going on the defensive.

Lisa described being worn down by daily notes and phone calls, which led her to question teachers' autism knowledge, saying, "I don't teach special ed. You tell me what to do. Don't be sending these damn notes home to me every day, telling me about what he did and blah blah this and blah blah that. He's autistic. You're a special ed teacher. Figure it out! I wanted a placement for him where people wouldn't be calling me and asking me a whole bunch of dumb questions." In turn, Lisa recalibrated the tensions and strategized on how she could help John's teachers better understand his behaviors. She decided to share John's love of '70s funk and R&B music with teachers because she noticed how music motivated, calmed, and held John's attention. John especially loved Rick James, Michael Jackson, and Prince. Lisa made CDs for his teachers to familiarize them with his musical selections, in the hopes that music would help regulate his body and improve classroom behaviors. In doing so, she recognized that his teachers are young White women who may not be familiar with the soundtrack of his life, thus, she took the initiative to ensure that teachers would understand John when he blurted out song lyrics. She also encouraged teachers to use music throughout the school day. The strategy was met with enthusiasm from John's teachers and served to connect school and home.

Schools can also build trust with Black mothers by demonstrating care and concern for their sons' well-being (Marchand et al., 2019). Several BAMs elaborated upon how caring communications and advocacy from school personnel built trust in tangible ways. For example, when Indigo's 17-year-old son Poobie prepared for a high-stakes statewide exam, school staff closely observed an uptick in anxiety-induced behaviors. The pressure of high-stakes testing caused Poobie to engage in biting and picking away at his nails and hands. Indigo shared how Poobie's school counselor reached out to express concerns about his mounting anxiety, saying, "I got a call from his counselor who said, 'Let me talk to you.' This woman called me at 8:30 that night and said, 'I watch your son. He worked hard, but he was completely just nervous and overwhelmed by it.'" The counselor's call helped confirm why Poobie's anxiety-ridden behaviors increased in the weeks leading up to the exam. Subsequently, the school appealed Poobie's grade, allowing him to receive credit under state education provisions for students with IEPs. The school then strategized with Indigo in preparation for another state test Poobie was slated to take during the summer. In doing so, the school acknowledged familial support in preparing Poobie for exams and told Indigo, "We know who your family is and we know that you're going to sit down and set up time to get him ready for the test." Indigo appreciated how the school recognized that a partnership was needed to ensure Poobie's academic success. She was confident that the school genuinely cared about Poobie.

BAMs' ability to trust schools was furthered when teachers shared effective autism techniques with them, demonstrating respect for Black mothers' roles in their sons' lives. School staff, in these instances, utilized strengths-based approaches when interacting with BAMs. Michelle shared how shortly after Sam's diagnosis she approached Sam's school staff with apprehension. "I couldn't trust him with just anybody." Despite her initial fears, Sam's earliest teachers and therapists taught her applied behavioral analysis (ABA) techniques and welcomed her into the classroom. Although she was new to autism, Sam's teachers respectfully engaged with her, placing Sam's well-being at the center of their interactions. Years later, she reflected upon how school staff proceeded, "[They] taught me the language, so I knew if I'm talking to a speech pathologist, I could talk about expressive and receptive language." The partnership yielded results across home and school settings, as Michelle structured Sam's homelife using ABA techniques. "The most important thing for me was for them to include me and for us to be partners in making decisions about interventions that they were going to try for him and to not unilaterally make decisions about him and not include me, that was critical for me and they saw that." Michelle cited Sam's earliest teachers and therapists as instrumental in raising her autism knowledge and empowering her future advocacy efforts.

When she moved upstate, Sam's classroom teachers were unfamiliar with ABA and sensory regulation, causing them to underestimate his skills. Her frustration grew and apprehension intensified as teachers called home daily with negative comments about Sam's classroom performance. Michelle was a single mother of two and was so unsettled by his schooling that she made the decision to remain unemployed until the situation stabilized. "When I first moved here, I couldn't even look for a job. I couldn't do anything until he was placed in the right school. I needed to be available. They called me every day to come up there and I would go and work with him. It wasn't that his behavior was extremely bad, but I think they just didn't know." Michelle then began to accompany Sam to school daily where her presence was met with resistance from the lead teacher, while his classroom aides were curious and receptive to learning ABA techniques.

> I came in and brought my little makeshift ABA kit to show them with the token reinforcement and the little pennies and things to show them the structure that my son needed in order for him to understand behavioral expectations and in order for them to even assess what he knew academically. It was a certain way. I had learned. I had learned from his teachers. They would watch me and watch the results I would get with him. They would say things like "oh wow, I didn't know he could do that."

Sam's original teachers imparted autism knowledge and empowered Michelle's assertiveness; she was positioned to instruct his new teachers on sensory techniques that benefited Sam and other students. In doing so, she challenged teachers to raise the bar of low expectations and demonstrated Sam's skill set. Michelle stated, "They assumed the glass was half full, that there wasn't anything going on up there. I would show them, there is. The teacher didn't think he knew his alphabet and then I just stood right up with the pointer and pointed and he's like, 'ABC.' Their mouths dropped open because they assumed because he didn't talk, or because he was crawling or climbing, that meant there was nothing going on upstairs. That wasn't the case."

Sam had sensory needs that Michelle realized were not being addressed. Thus, classroom visits allowed her to model sensory techniques for teachers. She recalled showing teachers techniques that may have looked strange but were sensory regulatory techniques that Sam's former occupational therapists taught her. She added, "Spending time on the floor with him and doing deep pressure activities and bringing in one of those exercise balls and doing different kinds of activities with him. They initially thought, 'Okay, that's odd,' but they didn't understand I was regulating his body to help him sit longer and help him attend and be able to listen in morning circle." Michelle's example further demonstrates that Black mothers want to work closely with schools to ensure educational outcomes are met. She was grateful for school collaborations that imparted autism techniques and broadened her autism knowledge. "I really appreciate all of the behavioral therapists and teachers and people that have helped me understand that there's a function to the behavior." Sam's new teachers integrated the techniques Michelle taught them, resulting in improved outcomes for Sam. Their ability to listen, engage, and learn resulted in greater trust and thus allowed her to pursue full-time employment.

Partnerships between autism providers and Black parents, as Pearson and Meadan (2021) argue, must serve to increase parental autism knowledge and empower families for advocacy. Similarly, participating BAMs were receptive to working with school staff for their sons' well-being. Openness to school-family partnerships occurred when mothers established trust with teachers and support staff when they were confident that schools were invested in positive outcomes for their sons. Trust served as the foundation for nonthreatening exchange of autism knowledge, advocacy skills, and pedagogical strategies. BAMs did not want to engage in power struggles but instead desired to share power with school staff to ensure positive outcomes for their sons. BAMs were aware of the contentious sociopolitical history of Black education, particularly that of Black boys, but they held high expectations for schools educating their sons.

Class Implications of BAMs' Advocacy

Participants were aware of how the experiences of White middle-class families are normalized in autism research and services yet determined that they would not be deterred (Broder-Fingert et al., 2020; Steinbrenner et al., 2022). For example, research attests to how White middle-class parents are empowered to challenge schools because they leverage resources, including knowledge of services, special education law, and familiarity with school systems (Harry, 2007; Kalyanpur et al., 2000). BAMs in this study, as previously noted, are all college-educated women with some participants holding advanced degrees. Black autism mothers' middle-class status and levels of education attainment, however, did not automatically buffer them from structural racism in health and education systems while advocating for autism services (Constantino et al., 2020; Durkin et al., 2017; Morgan & Stahmer, 2020; Stahmer et al., 2019; Straiton & Sridhar, 2022).

BAMs' educational levels and middle-class status did, however, contribute to their awareness of how social networks could be leveraged to navigate systems to access resources for their sons. Lisa explained, "I had the wherewithal to know to fight for him. I think some Black women especially, may not have that wherewithal, and I think that's what makes it difficult for us. Some of us have circumstances where, again, we're low-income, we don't have a supportive job, we may not have a supportive partner."

While social class provided insights on how to maneuver with school districts, it did not, however, mitigate challenging interactions with school staff. BAMs were very much aware that their advocacy occurred at the intersection of race, class, gender, and autism where privilege and oppression simultaneously occur (Collins & Bilge, 2016).

Middle-class status and higher education provided "the wherewithal" to understand the intricacies of special education, including the language, stakeholders, and laws. School psychologist Faith acknowledged her privilege and recognized that school systems marginalize many low-income parents of special needs students. Faith elaborated:

> So, it was just a matter of knowing those things, and being able to advocate, and push back, because, the funding piece is a driving force for schools, and if they can convince a parent that a student doesn't need a service, or that they just don't provide a service, or that it's not necessary, if a parent really doesn't know enough about the school system, then they're going to take the word of the CSE chairperson, and say, oh, okay. Take it off of the IEP, or, okay, I guess he won't have it. And I wasn't going for that.

Working in schools and conducting evaluations illuminated the role of funding in special education services, specifically, who gets services and who loses out on services.

Faith initially revealed little about her professional background to school personnel because she understood how social capital could shape perceptions of her advocacy efforts. She said, "They didn't learn that I was a school psychologist until his second-grade year . . . they just thought I was just always unhappy and pushing back on their recommendations. Once they learned that I was a school psychologist, that's when they started to understand that I knew special education law too, and so they weren't going to be able to just tell me anything, because if it didn't make sense, I was going to say something about it." Faith executed a three-pronged advocacy strategy: professional knowledge of law, developing insiders as allies, and classroom observations. Specifically, she gained the confidence of White mothers to find out how resources were differently availed to White families. In one instance, she advocated for whole-class music therapy, after learning from a White mother that it was available. While she still had to fight for services, Faith recognized that her positionality afforded opportunities that low-income Black families did not possess. The school recognized her as a formidable opponent because she expended social capital of special education law expertise and social networks, which equipped her to effectively navigate special education.

BAMs developed protective strategies to approach school leaders as they felt advocacy would be met with resistance by school leaders (Morgan & Stahmer, 2020). For example, Candi became an unoffical student of law and civics, as she diligently worked to learn special education laws while also introducing herself to key players in local and state education, and in the autism community. She also mentioned that her primary advocacy tool is asking, "Why?," pushing school staff to explain decision-making processes and urging them to think differently about solutions. In addition to battles around the CSE meeting table regarding Pappas's school placements, Candi engaged school staff on matters related to Pappas's safety, well-being, and self-esteem. In one instance, Pappas came home repeating a phrase a school employee leveled at him. Candi was infuriated to hear, "What are you, stupid," being used to address her son. Given Pappas's inability to directly name the school employee, Candi pulled out the school yearbook, which she regularly purchased for such instances, as a means of ensuring Pappas was well treated. She shared, "I found out a teaching assistant (TA) was saying this to him. 'What's the matter with you? What are you, stupid? Sit down.' We don't use that word. 'What are you, stupid? Sit down.' And he just kept saying it and saying it. So, I listened for a little while, and I said, 'Pappas, somebody saying that to you at school? Yes? Get the yearbook.'" Candi detailed how Pappas retrieved the yearbook and pointed to the photo of the offending staff member.

Evidence in hand, Candi called the school the next day and spoke with the vice principal to share details pertaining to the situation and vent her anger. She added, "Oh, I called him. I said, I told that vice principal, 'She got to go. She got to go.' I said, 'She either go, or I'm coming up there, and I'm going to break every bone in her face, because don't nobody call my baby stupid.' He's like, 'Mrs. Charles, we don't want you to do that.' Next time, I'm coming up there in my old sneakers with some Vaseline, no earrings, and my hair braided." Like other BAMs, Candi instinctively protected her son from mistreatment and invoked the expression "Vaseline, no earrings, and hair braided" to figuratively express her anger (Corbin et al., 2018; Smitherman, 1986).

As Black women, BAMs were aware that race and gender complicated the process of advocacy, with White teachers and school staff being confronted, challenged, and affronted by Black mothers. According to

Candi, BAMs have to advocate for their sons: "We go hard in the paint. [Schools] assume I'm angry."

"They Hate to See Me Coming Up to That School"

Study participants were conscious of how Black women are perceived as troublemaking, oppositional, and argumentative (Allen & White-Smith, 2018; Wilson Cooper, 2007; Zionts et al., 2003). As Beverly and other study participants described, Black mothers engage in a delicate balance of power with schools that necessitates readiness and protective stances. "They don't have no problems with me. We don't even go there no more. In the beginning, when they try you but I don't go there no more." While BAMs did not actively seek confrontation, they asserted themselves, developed strategies for advocacy, and established clear expectations of school staff.

BAMs recognized the high stakes of special education services and were emboldened to press districts for resources. Several participants expressed concerns about cuts to specialized services, like speech and occupational therapies, as their sons progressed through K–12 education. While districts moved to cut services due to budgetary constraints, BAMs pushed back because their sons' autism classification did not change. Beverly captured this point, saying, "They're trying to cut back on some of the stuff in his IEP, and that's where I step in at, but they always good for that. I guess I've been pretty lucky because I'm his mouthpiece." As his "mouthpiece," Beverly established clear expectations for school staff. She noted:

> As long as they don't mess with me and to be honest, these people here, they more scared of me than I am them. We get what we entitled to because I know my rights and my son's rights. The school is all White but I don't care. As long as they give my son the best education and they do. I don't have no problems. I've been fighting my whole life. Nothing is given to you. If you don't go after it. You're not going to get it. Somebody's going to get it but it ain't going to be you.

Beverly established a fault line with school staff, which if crossed would activate a more boisterous form of advocacy. According to Beverly, the school backed down from cutting Marvelous's services when she informed them, "I'm calling the superintendent. I'm getting ready to call Governor Cuomo up. I'll call the state reps. I'll do it. I'll send an email and put everybody on email. Yes indeed." As a Black mother in an overwhelmingly White district, Beverly recognized that her presence and knowledge of special education intimidated school staff, which she cleverly tapped into for hard-fought resource battles. Thus, she turned the negative perceptions back onto the school to benefit her son.

As Harry (2007) argues, Black parents want schools to be culturally competent, respectful, and committed to equitable practices. The absence of authentic collaboration based on these practices further contributes to gaps in special education services and outcomes for Black students. Karla's position as a school social worker reified these points and provided her insights on how to advocate for her two sons, 6-year-old Mikey and 11-year-old Andrew. In her professional experience, schools counted on parents opting out, not showing up to meetings, or simply going along with the suggestions of school officials (Kalyanpur et al., 2000). Karla believed this was the case with her attempts to advocate for Mikey, as teachers and school staff were not used to Black mothers strongly advocating at the CSE table. She added: "[School staff] are not happy that we were advocating for him, rather than letting them just place him where [they want to]. We question things, and push to get whatever he needs, and I don't think that they like that. I think they'd rather it be, parents who may not be as knowledgeable and don't advocate or don't show up at all, so that they can then make the decision they'd like to make." Karla saw firsthand how the special education annual meeting table functioned as an intersectional space with White school officials taking the position of all-knowing, thereby expecting Black mothers to cede knowledge of their children, discounting their voices.

While the tensions between schools and parents is not uncommon in special education, the intersection of race and gender exacerbated differences in teachers' professional knowledge and BAMs' parental knowledge. BAMs of school-aged sons collectively spoke of adversarial interactions between them and White school staff, primarily White women. For example, Karla believed school officials were working behind the scenes to introduce an additional diagnosis for Mikey after severe classroom meltdowns. According to Karla, school staff were not clinically trained to determine an additional diagnosis, but she grew concerned: "Some of the staff members there may not say it to me, but it's almost as though, we're at times being told it could be something else and not autism because Mikey can show aggression."

Similarly, Kiara believed that school staff "don't like to see [her] coming," because she is not afraid to challenge assumptions about her son. She shared how, in one instance, Johnathan's teacher attempted to diagnose him with depression and anxiety. Kiara took great offense and immediately checked the teacher, as she reminded the woman that Johnathan's autism manifests in self-talk. "You see him going to his mind and watch his video game and watch his TV show. You see him laugh at his own jokes. That's not depression and anxiety." Kiara believes she simply advocates for Johnathan because it needs to be done. "I don't do it aggressively and I don't do it in a mean manner, but you're not going to speak death over my child and you're not going to just say anything." Mistrust in this instance stemmed from school staff making judgments outside professionally prescribed roles, judgments that Kiara believed could further stigmatize her son.

Kiara's adversarial interactions with school personnel heightened as she advocated over the course of several months for a one-to-one aide. Here again, conflicts surfaced between Kiara's parental insights on Johnathan and teachers' professional knowledge, which also increased her suspicions of racial discrimination (Lareau & Horvat, 1999). The battle for an aide waged while Johnathan's behaviors flared until, finally, CSE members agreed that he needed an aide to help with transitions, thereby decreasing intense behaviors. Kiara commented, "Hmmm, I find that funny. I thought about that 3 months ago. They didn't listen to me." Arguably, parents engage in battles with district officials over classroom aides due to cost, but Kiara believes that the skirmishes are also due to reticence and a refusal to validate the standpoint knowledge of Black autism mothers.

Based on the narratives of BAMs, school staff interpret BAMs' advocacy as a personalized racism accusation, when mothers are advocating for special education resources (Morgan & Stahmer, 2020). As Karla stated, "I think that some people don't expect me, as a Black woman, to advocate for a child." BAMs provided multiple examples of how school staff interpreted Black women's advocacy as a direct affront to them. Consequently, BAMs shared how White school personnel responded negatively, resulting in a focus on BAMs and not their sons. Said otherwise, Black mothers' advocacy was negatively perceived as a threat, causing entanglements that diverted attention away from sons and generated consuming hostility toward BAMs.

In the case of Faith, school staff labeled her as a "problem mom." Following a CSE meeting in which Faith fought for continued occupational therapy, she learned that her son's occupational therapist spoke disparagingly of her in front of school personnel, who then informed Faith. She was grateful to learn precisely what the occupational therapist thought of her. She recalled the incident:

> So, I got wind that the occupational therapist labeled me as a problem mom, because I had pushed back on her dropping the service for my child. And when we got to the meeting, I called her out about it. She did a lot of backpedaling. I basically said, "So, I'm aware that you have expressed to the vice principal that I'm a problem mom, because I don't want you to discontinue a service when my son is obviously still showing an area of need." And then she started saying, "Well, I didn't say that you were a problem mom. I just said that there was some pushback about the service, and blah, blah, blah." And I'm like, "I'm not here to debate you about whether or not you said it, because I believe you said it, but at this point, I just need you to understand that you're not going to just push my child off the table like he's nothing or disregard him. If I'm telling you he needs this service, he needs this service."

Here again, this incident highlights how a staff member's dislike of Faith manifested in name calling and distracted the focus away from her son. As a result of the conversation, Faith reported that the principal asked the occupational therapist to step outside the room, where the therapist was reprimanded.

"I Feel Threatened": A Teacher Calls the Police

This chapter would be remiss without a deeper consideration of BAMs' motherwork, that is, the ways in which Black women mother at the intersection of race, class, and gender. Motherwork is contextualized in a racist society that positions Black mothers as deviant, uncaring, and disengaged from their children's well-being (Wilson Cooper, 2007). To the contrary, Black women's motherwork directly confronts oppressive systems for the sake of nurturing Black children's physical, psychological, and economic well-being. Black women, like those featured in this study, understand that hegemonic forces work against the interests of Black children in special education and, thus, stand prepared to advocate for services and equitable resources. Thus, BAMs approached motherwork with seriousness, intentionality, and urgency because their sons' fates rested squarely upon their shoulders.

Motherwork, as demonstrated by study participants, also entailed protecting sons from physical danger and psychological harm. BAMs' protective stances were especially heightened due to the vulnerability of children on the autism spectrum, some of whom cannot verbalize when hurt or harm befalls them. Black autism mothers fought to protect their sons' humanity because the world can be cruel and lack understanding of autism-related behaviors. It should be noted that Black women incur the cost of motherwork in added stress, anxiety, health concerns, and other psychological manifestations of racial trauma and fatigue (Bryant-Davis & Ocampo, 2005; Corbin et al., 2018).

In this section, I take a deeper dive into BAMs' advocacy, focusing exclusively on Thelma's motherwork. Her narrative serves as a case within a case, as she directly challenged and confronted school authorities about her son's mistreatment. Readers hear from Thelma's 14-year-old son, Elijah, in his own words as he sought to make sense of bullying at the hands of classmates. Thelma's case provides insights into why Black women engage in motherwork, as she challenged Elijah's marginalization and invisibilization by school personnel (McDonald, 1997). The narrative also provides insights into motherwork behind the scenes—how Black mothers' protective love functions to rebuild children's self-worth and instill hope (Chapman & Bhopal, 2013; Collins, 1994; Wilson Cooper, 2007).

Sacrifices for Special Education Services

Thelma grew up in Upstate New York, but several years ago she decided to relocate to Texas for better economic and educational opportunities for her two sons, Elijah and his 7-year-old brother Solomon. Upon her arrival, she quickly learned the landscape of district-based autism resources and realized she needed to move yet again, into a White suburban district to receive better services for her boys. She focused on "finding the best fit and special ed options for them." Thelma continued: "We packed up and moved to a different district where we had option one, two, and option three has two teachers and a pear tree. I was a mother who put it out on the line for them. I appreciate that districts have to try with staffing and all, but that's not my baby's problem. I need him in a safe calm place where he can function." She weathered autism services in a large urban district but encountered uncertainties in staffing, autism services, and availability of placements. Instead, she chose to "follow the services" to gain access to steadier staffing and programming, noting that children on the spectrum do not respond well to daily environmental changes; they thrive on routine.

Schooling at the intersection of race, class, and gender often forces Black mothers to weigh the impact of school choice on the children's educational, socioemotional, and racial development (Allen & White-Smith, 2018; Chapman & Bhopal, 2013; Wilson Cooper, 2007).

Thelma realized that transitioning into a suburban environment also meant a trade-off in racially/ethnically diverse curriculum, student demographics, and social class. With a focus on autism services, she rationalized the trade-off, saying, "I don't send them to school for Blackness; they get that at home and the church. I send them to school to learn and be safe. I love my community, but I had to put all that aside to take care of my boys." She realized that moving into a White district would introduce additional stressors around race, class, and gender.

Elijah enjoyed school and thrived in technology-rich, highly structured classroom environments. He received classroom supports but was placed in general education because of his academic strengths. Over the course of several months, however, Thelma recounted how Elijah began to withdraw and resisted attending school because he experienced daily bullying by the same group of students. His behaviors made sense only when she stumbled across a handwritten letter buried deep in his book bag. In the letter, Elijah drew upon vocabulary learned in English class; he referred to himself as the protagonist and labeled his tormentors as the antagonist. The letter is reprinted here with both Thelma and Elijah's permission and reads as follows:

> I know, I got in trouble all the time because I should've been a nice men today. I became a "mean men" every single day while I was punished for all my actions. At [this] Middle School, none of these 8th grade girls are being nice at all! They're mean girls. I have to play a role in education so I can become a protagonist person, not an antagonist person. I should be cast as a good man and a protagonist Elijah Fox all the time via playing the role I'm best known for. I have to start doing things for myself all the time forever. I should get focused and learn things important all the time forever too. I would have to act like

professional people, because I'm getting into high school and into college for some support and all that, high school is for big kids like teenagers. I knew better than that if it's not true. ABC Middle School shows crazy people. ABC Middle school is a bad place, showing crazy people, inappropriate people, stupid 6–8th graders, and antagonist people. NONE! None of these 6–8th people are being very nice at all! I'm so sick of going to ABC Middle school because ABC Middle School shows stupid, antagonist and inappropriate people from 6-th forever! I am not ever get back together!

On the surface, the letter provides some insights on Elijah, a young man conscientious of his behaviors, with a recognition of how his shifting school behaviors categorize him as a "mean man" or "antagonist." He profoundly wants to be a "good man," a "protagonist person" but the actions of classmates, and lack of action by school officials, have led him to a self-described loner state. The frightening milieu of mean girls and boys ratchets the middle schooler's angst, leading him to label the antagonists as "crazy." He looks forward to high school and college for more support and more mature classmates.

After his mother coaxed him into sharing more details, Elijah filled in the missing pieces of the story: he was subjected to classmates pushing, throwing items at him, stealing items out of his bag, and ridiculing him. Elijah then shared how he wrote the letter in response to multiple incidents of bullying and told his mother that he felt alone during the school day as he traversed the hallways. Thelma was incensed with the "antagonists," but more so with school staff who failed to notify her regarding the bullying.

Subsequently, Thelma reached out to teachers and administrators via email with no response from school officials. She made the decision to keep Elijah at home, out of concern for his safety and mounting anxiety. Thelma emailed the school daily to report Elijah absent and commented, "He was sick, I didn't lie—sick and tired of the school. I would send a note in every day. We didn't want any other student to catch what Elijah had. They didn't have enough police officers if the kids all caught what he had." She opted instead to school him at home and sent yet another impassioned email, but this time to district senior staff, totaling over 50 people. Finally, after 18 days, the school contacted her regarding the bullying.

The School Meeting

What followed was a heated meeting at the school with Thelma, Elijah's father, Micah, Elijah's teachers, principal, and district-level special education leaders. Thelma and Micah hired an independent special education advocate who possessed over 25 years of advocacy experience. Although the couple incurred a cost to hire the advocate, the specialist's presence lowered her anxiety and, as she headed into the meeting, enabled her to maintain her focus. She stated, "I might have been in jail without the advocate. It's still unclear what happened because my child cannot verbalize it. Assault, attempt to rob him of clothes, money, phone, gym shorts taken. I had terrible thoughts on how the gym shorts were taken." The meeting was recorded by the advocate with full knowledge and permission of district officials and Thelma shared the recording with me. She warned me in advance of listening to the recording, "It's a powerful clip. That clusterfuck was documented! Their behaviors and responses documented!" The district officials postured defensively and never fully answered the question regarding why Thelma was not notified about the bullying incidents. She described how during the course of the meeting, it was important for her to represent Elijah: "With an autistic child, you have to lose yourself a little bit and walk in their shoes. I had to become my child. I'm a protagonist man and they're making me an antagonist man. He had to be someone other than himself."

At a critical point in the meeting, Elijah's classroom teacher can be heard sobbing, to which Thelma pointedly remarked, "You don't get the right to cry. I cried every day for 14 years. You had him in your class and failed to contact me, so you do not have the right to cry." The teacher left the room in response to Thelma's refute of her tears. A few moments later, the teacher returned but was accompanied by a police officer, the school's resource officer, who is heard entering the room and introducing himself. The teacher called the police officer after Thelma's rebuke. In a moment straight out of DiAngelo's (2018) analysis of White fragility, Elijah's teacher weaponized her tears and personalized the incident after being placed on the defensive. With the focus shifted off Elijah, the teacher recentered the heated racialized discussion back on her, leveraging law enforcement to sustain her innocence. Law enforcement further reified the underlying belief that Black mothers are aggressive, dangerous, and deserving of silencing.

Instead of listening to the message, the teacher interpreted Thelma's words as a threat of violence toward her, thereby criminalizing Thelma and dismissing her advocacy. The issue of Elijah's bullying was left unresolved even though Thelma expressed in advance her desire for additional supports to ensure Elijah's safety across the day. Thelma later learned that the teacher called the officer into the meeting saying that she "felt threatened" by Thelma and Elijah's father, who incidentally towers at 6 ft. 10 in. Thelma described the experience: "[It was an] outer body experience. The cop escorted me, father, child, and advocate off campus but the perpetrators are still there in class in my child's gym shorts. I felt like everyone should have been in cuffs. But people didn't give a damn. It was all about them." Here again, the intersection of race, class, gender, and autism resulted in the silencing and dismissing of a Black autism mother from the decision-making table. Not only was Thelma silenced, but law enforcement was leveraged to muzzle and invisibilize a mother who sought answers and solutions to her Black son being bullied in a largely White school district. The sudden introduction of law enforcement immediately ended the meeting, with the officer escorting the family and their advocate off campus.

"I Gave Him His Power Back"

In the aftermath, the district agreed to admit Elijah to an exclusive high school, located in an upper-class neighborhood. While she believes the school will be a good fit for him, Thelma realized she still needed to reacclimate Elijah to school, not only due primarily to his mistrust of school as a whole but, specifically, teachers and other students. She feared that his spirit was battered and noticed that physical reminders of school, like his book bag, frightened him. "He didn't even want to open the book bag." Thelma describes how she tapped into her son's fears and attempted to spiritually alleviate his fears by cleansing his book bag, as the bag was a source of anxiety and the target of bullying. In doing so, she believed that BAMs must demonstrate life lessons to their sons in direct yet spiritual ways:

> You gotta paint the picture when you're a Black autistic momma. We had to do it in the bathroom and take each piece out to help him understand it is okay to go into your book bag, so he is not afraid. I had to wash it so that all the meanness, evil,

Education at the Intersection of Race, Class, Gender, and Autism | 115

violation, hands that touched it will be washed away so it will be like new. He told me to put extra detergent on it, I said, "Okay baby." Those people wanted me to get my extra sneakers, Vaseline, and go whoop somebody ass 'bout my baby. But I gave him his power back.

Thelma believes she stays ready to battle for her kids and does admit to getting loud when the safety of her children is in question. "I was fact checking. Pulling cards. Fake news all up in that motherfucker. I got heated and loud 'cause you don't hear me tho'." Thelma's anger was heightened after it was revealed during the meeting that Elijah's tormentors had additional plans to bully and harass him. Given the deleterious meeting conclusion, it is important to contextualize Thelma's anger as resistance to the school's minimization of Elijah's bullying. As Corbin et al. (2018) described, Thelma engaged in Black women's talk, a racial and gendered discursive resistance to social injustices. Thus, her comments functioned to empower protective instincts and defiance of school personnel's stereotypes (Houston, 2000; Smitherman, 1986).

Chapter Summary

Black autism mothers, like many Black mothers, approached schools apprehensively, because they are fully cognizant of how schools position Black mothers as difficult, aggressive, ignorant, and uncaring (Wilson Cooper, 2007). To the contrary, participating mothers sought collaborative school relationships built on a foundation of mutual respect, equity, and humane treatment of their sons. Several mothers provided insights on positive home–school collaborations though the exchange of autism expertise on a level plain—schools shared autism behavioral techniques and BAMs shared expert knowledge of sons. Mothers with positive school relationships appreciated judgment-free interactions, cultural competence, and in-school advocacy on behalf of their sons (Harry, 2007). Black autism mothers, although cautious, were open to school partnerships and illuminated the intentional work of schools required for collaboration.

Mothers remained on alert for racial offenses and developed strategies to confront school officials. Establishing clear lines of delineation of acceptable interactions was important to some BAMs, playing upon and flipping stereotypes of Black mothers back on school staff. Mothers identified staff members willing to serve as allies, providing inside information on untrustworthy staff who worked against their sons' best interests. Such staff were key in mothers developing counterstrategies to proposed autism service reductions. BAMs gleaned information from other autism parents to fortify arguments for sustained or additional autism resources. When White mothers boasted about autism resources, one BAM listened intently and leveraged the information to receive equitable services. Information shared by White mothers provided yet another example of how power and privilege underscore the distribution of autism resources in schools.

The motherwork of autism advocacy directly challenges systemic practices that harm Black children. BAMs felt justified in their advocacy efforts, no matter how schools perceived them, as they understood the connection between advocacy, interventions, and positive outcomes for Black boys in special education. As middle-class Black women, participants were profoundly aware of their positionality—the dichotomy of class privilege and oppression. BAMs expended social capital (Lareau & Horvat, 1999) and simultaneously acknowledged that education and professional status allowed them to maneuver and advocate in ways not afforded to low-income Black autism mothers.

Chapter 6

Black Is the New Autism

BAMs and Autism Representation

Representation matters. I grew up in an era where it was unusual to see Black people on TV. I can remember getting excited whenever I saw Black people on prime time TV in guest star roles or even as extras—excitement that triggered rapid-fire phone calls to my cousins across the city: "Turn to 10 . . . it's Black people on TV." I devoured weekly *Jet* and monthly *Ebony* magazines within hours of them landing in our mailbox. Representation matters.

I felt the same way in the years immediately following Caleb's diagnosis. I looked online to learn more about autism resources, especially those related to schooling and specific topics like sensory diets and the Individuals with Disabilities Education Act. Those searches left me wondering, where were the moms who looked like me? Where were the kids who looked like Caleb? I got to the point of tuning out because the narrative was the same—quit your job, make autism your life's focus, move to a better district, and so on. Why was autism parenting so narrowly interpreted?

The politics of representation is more than just seeing Black mothers and sons though—it's about seeing the possibilities of how Black mothers arrange their lives. The possibilities of how Black mothers balance their children's autism care with work, family, and self-care. What happens at the intersection of being Black, middle class, working full-time, and mothering a son with autism? What happens when all those identities collide? That's what I needed to hear, see, and feel. Representation is about disrupting essentialized notions about autism. It was as if we did not exist or were not important.

Fast-forward a few years, and now Black autism families and Black autism voices can be found across social media platforms. Autism Mocha Moms, Autism in Black, the Color of Autism Foundation, and the Mocha Autism Network all provide resources for Black families in culturally grounded ways. I follow a Black single autism dad who chronicles he and his boy's daily activities navigating the big city. He uses the platform to share his moments of triumph, nagging doubts, and love for his son. I appreciate reading his posts because he is rewriting the narrative of Black fathers and autism. Then there's the young lady who speaks her truth of being a Black woman with autism in a society where she does not "fit" stereotypical representations of autistic youth. I recently even saw a Black mom and her son on a fast-food restaurant commercial where she thanked a Black female employee who regularly interacted with her autistic son. Mom emphasized that her son was "seen." The respectful interactions of the restaurant employee with the young Black male meant something to that Black mother—her child was seen. He was heard. Being seen means something. Being heard means something. Establishing one's voice means something.

A few years ago, Caleb participated in a writing workshop led by students from a local university. Writing was introduced as a therapeutic device, allowing participants to express themselves and share their interests. The workshop triggered a notable change in Caleb—he started writing his story. Caleb now uses writing to self-regulate and tap into his creative side. He has filled countless notebooks with dystopian tales about a modern world in which mankind's survival hinges upon the forces of good and evil engaged in epic gory battles. There's a hero, an antagonist, lots of fighting, chivalry, and at least one half-dressed hot girl. (His stories include hot girls because after all, he says, "I'm a guy, Mom." I replied, "Yeah, but we gotta talk about misogyny . . ."). He finds his stories deliriously entertaining as I've watched him smile, laugh, and giggle while writing. His story settings shift across remote areas of Asia, the South Pacific, Central America, and sub-Saharan locations. His heroes identify with causes of social justice, fighting against unjust imprisonment and enslavement of colored peoples. The stories always have a clear-cut sense of right and wrong.

The battles in some of the stories are a bit much and make me uncomfortable. So, one day I asked him, "Why is there so much violence in these stories?" He replied, "Well Mom, I write stories that I like. I wanna save people and fight the bad guys. My characters get to do the things I want to do." I was so struck by his words—Caleb recognizes that he has a voice with valuable social critiques, but it's easier to do so in a fictionalized world where he always comes out on top. He writes himself into existence, creating a world where his actions matter—he's saving lives and leading his people to victory against oppressive forces. In one story,[1] for instance, historical figures like Huey P. Newton, Nelson Mandela, and Caesar Chavez were used to describe a political figure dedicated to his people. The story's hero then "guides lost souls with a presence like a Harriet Tubman using a lantern to guide people to freedom and beyond. Truly a man with a scar on his face is a man who has character." Caleb has a scar on his face.

I am Caleb's mom and I see you, son. You are my hero.

Autism parents of this generation, unlike previous generations, have access to countless sources of autism information via in-person and online autism support groups, autism advocacy organizations, and autism research centers. Social media platforms abound with autism parents posting about their advocacy efforts and day-to-day experiences parenting children with autism. Parents can now more readily access autism research and even connect with researchers from across the globe. Autism information is accompanied by imagery of who autism impacts and what autism looks like, contributing to a broader narrative of an autism community. Autism cultural spaces include physical locations and online sites dedicated to autism prevention, treatment, and education. In addition to autism care providers and clinicians, the interests of autism families shape broader autism agendas with nonprofit organizations, corporate sponsorships, and organized advocacy and legislative lobbying efforts seeking to improve the lives of individuals with autism. Moreover, autism cultural spaces are also social locations where, unlike in previous eras, parents' autism knowledge prevails and challenges that of researchers and medical professionals (Douglas, 2013).

Autism cultural spaces are punctuated by a distinct representation of motherhood, where images of White mothers battling autism through sacrifice of careers and outside social interests abound (Angell & Solomon,

---

[1]. Caleb sends me his stories via text messages and in Google Docs.

2017; DeWolfe, 2015; Douglas, 2013). For example, a recent financial planning company commercial depicts a White mother who accesses capital needed to start a business to provide employment for her son. White autism mothers are the face of autism and invoke images of warriorlike tenacity while battling autism head-on (Chivers Yochim & Silva, 2013). White autism warrior mothers, as conveyed by autism cultural imagery, contest the male-dominated medical profession, which had for years labeled autism mothers as "refrigerator mothers" and discredited mothers' experiential knowledge (Bettelheim, 1959, 1967; Douglas, 2014; Kanner, 1943).

Observing an online autism event posting, Douglas (2013) described White autism mothers' warrior stances, noting that these mothers stand "ready": "White and female with long brown or blonde hair stand posed in a line, most angled in and toward one another, one facing away. Their stance is wide, like they are ready for action. They appear slim and 'fit' and stand tall, their necks long, bare shoulders thrown back. No one smiles. Those mothers who are actively engaged in the battle for services, in the case of the warrior mother images, are white women" (p. 173). Good deeds aside, imagery of autism warrior mothers must be examined as purveyors of a particular kind of autism mothering predicated upon exclusivity—a special group of White autism mothers who are empowered by social standing, wealth, and education to combat autism through charitable work. While images of White autism mothers control autism narratives, Black autism expert (and autism mother) Diana Paulin warns that such representations must be problematized, as they function to the detriment of White women while simultaneously excluding Black women. She states, "Even though there are terrible problems with these tropes, including punishing representations of motherhood, Black women are excluded even from that. In these representations, these Black women are trying to find a place for themselves in these autism stories and they're like 'I can't even be a refrigerator mother!'" (Paulin, as cited in Rodas, 2021, p. 123). Similarly, participants in this study challenge race-neutral autism narratives and respond to questions regarding the presence of Black autism mothers in autism cultural spaces.

This chapter takes up the question of Black mothers' presence in autism cultural spaces and challenges the prevailing idea that autism is race and class neutral. To the contrary, Black autism mothers in this study were cognizant of how Whiteness is central to autism cultural spaces. The cases of two mothers are examined to illuminate how Black mothers "show up" in autism spaces populated primarily by White autism mothers. The centering of Whiteness in autism spaces challenged Black autism mothers to create autism spaces within Black cultural settings. These efforts were not always met with acceptance, as some participants recounted resistance within Black churches. Ever aware of misguided notions of race neutrality in autism, the chapter concludes with Black mothers advising autism clinicians and providers on culturally responsive practices.

The Autism Cultural Scene

Langan (2011) argues that no one group of parents can speak for all autism parents and posits that a multitude of parental voices bring varied experiential knowledge to bear on autism parenting. She maintains that autism parents, mothers in particular, play an important role in challenging assumptions about the condition and raising public awareness of autism, saying:

> Parents do not speak with one voice: parental voices in relation to autism have always been diverse and have often been discordant. Parents have contributed to these discussions from a number of distinct perspectives. Some speak as parents, claiming no particular expertise other than their personal experience as parents. Others speak as lay experts, having painstakingly acquired expertise, often in areas of science and medicine, through personal research and study (facilitated in recent years by the internet). Others still speak as parents with particular academic or professional expertise. (p. 194)

Parental voices have been galvanized by the exchange of parental expertise on social media platforms, as one study participant shared her experiences posting and maintaining an active presence in an online autism support group.

Most study participants did not actively seek out or participate in autism cultural spaces due to a variety of reasons. BAMs were cognizant that organizations led by White women likely maintained autism agendas focused on the needs of White middle-class families, as people of color rarely occupied seats at the leadership table. Socializing in autism spaces with White mothers took energy that most BAMs were not interested in exerting, as they remained focused on creating and maintaining Black cultural connections. Participants did not view autism and race as dichotomous, but they were cognizant of how autism cultural spaces can prove unwelcoming for Black mothers and families. Two study participants, Marley and Kendra, did, however, seek out autism cultural spaces with a regional organization and an online autism parenting discussion group.

Forty-year-old Kendra was the lone BAM who actively participated in an online support group; she was encouraged to join by clinicians and other mothers interested in her pharmacy background and experiences raising twin boys on the autism spectrum. Mother to 7-year-old twins affectionately known as Papa Smurf and Lil Man, Kendra developed personal and professional knowledge of Medicaid and willingly shared information with focus group members, especially on issues pertaining to insurance coverage of toileting supplies. She described her participation in the group: "I'm learning a lot through the autism group, Facebook group. People post questions a lot about everything . . . , with some medication questions to having issues with the pull-ups. I'm an expert at that. A lot of times they get referred to me." Because her contributions were valued and sought out, Kendra enjoyed participating and helping other parents navigate the complicated maze of Medicaid benefits. While her expertise was highly valued by the social media group, Kendra's position as a pharmacist in a Black and Latino urban community motivated her to share her Medicaid expertise with pharmacy customers. She spoke to this point, adding,

> I've spent the better part of more than a year really learning how to build or redo [our Medicaid application]. I'm actually contracted with the approved contractor through state Medicaid. I've gotten several, I've gotten probably a dozen families referred to me for that. Then I also, of course I do those two, my two little people. Even before I started doing my two little people, I was already doing a few people just in my customer base. I dug deeper.

Kendra positioned herself to learn about Medicaid benefits and shared her professional expertise with her Black and Latino customer base. While Kendra is to be commended for navigating multiple autism cultural spaces, she leveraged her professional expertise to maneuver in autism cultural spaces.

Marley, an energetic 35-year-old, longed for connections to other autism families. The strains of mothering two children, one of whom has autism, left her feeling increasingly isolated and "trying to find a community that I feel like I fit in." She wanted to learn from other mothers and share her own experiences; she wanted to be in community with others raising children with autism. Marley became aware of activities of the local chapter of a national autism organization regularly hosted at their suburban offices. The organization's draw, according to Marley, was the wide range of recreational, informational, and training activities, including summer camps. The organization provided programming at a direct cost to families. While the programmatic offerings appealed to Marley, the organization's public images gave her some pause, as their social media and website did not feature Black families. The local autism grapevine also confirmed her unease that very few families of color participated in the organization's programming. This raised some concerns, but she remained undeterred and decided to give the organization a chance in the hopes that a shared interest in autism would allay concerns of an unwelcoming environment.

After attending a few functions at the organization's suburban location, Marley decided that she was done; she vowed never to attend any functions hosted by the organization again, explaining, "I don't feel that I fit in with [the organization]. I think it's a little bit too White and I don't want to go [to that suburb] all the time." In retrospect, she reflected on how the location would prove challenging to families without transportation, as the facility was hard to access via public transportation. The location was convenient only to those families within close proximity. Aside from these concerns, Marley was also bothered by how the programming was cost prohibitive, which she believed further contributed to the preponderance of White families. She clarified her feelings:

> The reason I don't feel comfortable with [the organization] is because the majority of the mothers and the children are White. I think it's frustrating because while we have something in common, there's also something in common we don't have and [they] don't get it. It was birthed out of the suburban community which from a financial aspect, that they have a little bit more of a disposable income and are able to do things. The organization, it's not cheap, it's not cheap for a 7-week class.

> Being able to come up with $300 is not cheap, and I thought we were middle class. Their middle class is not my middle class!

The common bond of autism was not enough to keep Marley engaged in the organization's activities, as cost, distance, and racial isolation led to her disengagement. As Marley highlights, the organization's "birth" story did not entail a consideration of how families outside that community and families of color could access services.

The following summer, Marley found a welcoming space in a grant-funded project sponsored by an urban school district in partnership with a local university. Similar to recommendations by Maye et al. (2022), community partnerships should collaboratively engage Black families with researchers and service providers in culturally responsive ways. Marley participated in a program that targeted Black and Latino families and, according to Marley, provided an engaging and welcoming space to share experiential knowledge and learn about autism communication strategies. She believed the program was effective because

> They offered quarterly classes, and they brought in folks from the outside. They didn't consider themselves experts, but they brought in folks from different autistic camps to be able to tell us about this and what this looks like and the age requirement. They understood our concerns as parents with autistic kids, especially those who don't know how to communicate well. Being able to have staff that truly they can trust . . . they helped us and our children be able to express themselves.

Common interests in autism do not serve as an automatic rallying point for Black mothers seeking support, as Black mothers' positionality is shaped by continued injustice at the intersection of race, class, and gender. Injustice is personal for Black autism mothers and frames how BAMs show up or present themselves in community-based autism spaces. Black women's positionality may also contribute to resistance to joining autism organizations with agendas built around the needs of White middle-class women. While parental expertise has shaped public perceptions of autism and raised awareness across social media, schools, and clinical settings, the exercise of expertise has served to benefit White autism mothers (Eyal & Hart, 2010). Parental expertise does not, however, occur in a social vacuum as expertise is derived, developed, and shared at the intersection of race, class, gender, and autism.

BAMs Kendra and Marley provide examples of how BAMs show up, or present in autism cultural spaces. Kendra persisted and sustained involvement with an online autism support group while Marley tried her hand at attending events hosted by an autism organization. While both had different outcomes, their experiences speak to Black autism mothers' willingness to engage in overwhelmingly White autism cultural spaces with different modalities. The online support group provided a social buffer not afforded by in-person interactions, as Kendra freely shared her professional, educational, and personal expertise with the group. Autism parents and professionals posted questions and responded. Kendra shared that she became known for helping parents navigate Medicaid benefits, positioning her as an expert in the group. Her sustained involvement in the group yielded expert status, validation, and respect.

Conversely, the modality of in-person engagement with White mothers and families at an autism organization led Marley to disengage. While she sought the emotional support and comfort of being in community with other autism mothers, Marley approached with a measured dose of optimism tempered by a lifetime of interactions with White women in predominately White spaces. She entered the space fully expecting the stressors Black women face when interacting with White women in clinical, educational, and workspaces; Black women daily navigate racial and gendered hegemony (DiAngelo, 2018). Thus, for mothers like Marley, the work of in-person engagement in White-dominated autism cultural spaces did not yield the desired outcomes of emotional support and expanded autism expertise.

Her desire to join an autism community outweighed her trepidations of being invisibilized and unheard by White autism mothers. In-person engagement evokes vulnerability to judgment and simultaneously requires mothers to feel safe, welcomed, and respected among other autism mothers. Despite her efforts to engage, the experience left Marley feeling like a social and economic outsider. The organization's atmosphere created a barrier to involvement and prevented Marley from gaining what she needed: a welcoming and nurturing autism community. Marley's account of the urban organization provides a counterpoint to her experiences with the suburban organization. She actively participated in the group, sharing her expertise while learning from other families and professionals. The contrasting experiences speak to how organizations that exclusively serve the interests of White families lose out on the experiences and social and economic contributions of Black autism families.

Representations of autism as an exclusively White condition is not due to a lack of interest on the part of Black autism mothers. To the contrary, the cases of Kendra and Marley challenge the misnomer that race, class, and gender are of no concern in autism cultural spaces. The proliferation of White mothers as the public face of autism is not reflective of Black autism mothers' lack of interest in learning, sharing, and communing with other autism families. Instead, lack of representation results from structural inequities, with White mothers creating social and economic opportunities around advocacy (Douglas, 2013; Langan, 2011). As demonstrated in the next section, Black autism mothers are seeking wholeness: they want autism spaces that fully embrace Black cultural connectedness.

Black Autism Mothers Creating Autism Cultural Spaces

Although the mothers in this study describe themselves as occupying the margins of the autism community because they did not actively participate in formalized autism organizations, the choice to opt out of existing organizations did not leave them disempowered. For other Black autism mothers, autism cultural spaces were synonymous with Black cultural spaces, as mothers needed to maintain cultural connections to ensure wellness and personal fulfillment. These mothers found it difficult and unnecessary to separate themselves from Black cultural spaces, such as Black churches, even if it meant fighting to create autism spaces in their respective congregations. Social and cultural connections with Black communities was important, and BAMs were willing to teach others about autism to ensure their sons benefited from participation in community settings.

Two BAMs formed their own nonprofit organizations to fill a void of services for Black autism families and others living in urban areas. Candi's small nonprofit targeted families of color across her region. As her organization grew, Candi began to leverage social media to reach families of color in other regions of the state, with invitations to various events. Ending social isolation among families of color through family-themed autism events became the focus of Candi's nonprofit. For example, during the data collection stage of this study, Candi's organization hosted a morning activity focused on art and crafts and simultaneous building of social networks of Black autism families, which is fundamental to her mission. The organization also regularly plays host to a support group that targets Black autism families.

Candi is serious about the organizational mission of empowering Black parents to share their experiences of rearing children on the spectrum, as she realized most would not join White-led support groups. Through her experiences interacting with other Black parents in community settings, Candi believed the time was right to engage in deep, meaningful discussions that would serve to empower Black autism parents. Black autism parents' fears of vulnerability, she believed, limited their ability to connect with each other's joys and pains:

> We talk about it, but we clean it up. Don't clean it up. Tell me. Yeah. I give them the raw and they look at me like . . . and then sometimes with some of them, I see like the melt. . . . This one lady, I said one thing to her, and we wind up standing in the laundromat for 45 minutes! When I got in my car, I said, "Okay, Lord. You sent me there, because she needed to talk about that." [She] started being more real with me, because sometimes I feel like [Black autism mothers] don't want to be bothered with each other. Because I was reaching out for her, for the last 4 years.

According to Candi, Black autism parents needed a judgment-free space to share their stories to support and empower each other. Black autism parents are already marginalized in autism spaces, but as Candi articulated, they further isolate themselves from each other. Her mission was to build upon a shared cultural foundation to provide much-needed support for each other.

Based upon her experiences addressing her son Dwayne's social-emotional and leadership development, Sarah became disenchanted with his school's inability to simultaneously address his personal and academic development. This concern led her to not only pursue a master's degree in special education but to start a nonprofit organization geared to developing social-emotional and academic skills in adolescents on the spectrum. While Sarah did not directly target her mission to an exclusive Black autism population, her nonprofit's mission is raising self-esteem in teens with autism through STEAM (science, technology, engineering, arts, and math) programming. Situated in her predominantly Black and

Latino school district, Sarah's organization stemmed from her "frustration with the lack of quality services for children with special needs, quality services that you can afford because they really don't bloody well exist." Thus far, her foundation has provided after-school robotics programming for elementary age kids with plans to scale up to middle and high school. The program is self-sustaining as participating teachers are now training other teachers in the program curriculum. Sarah hosts yearly fundraising activities including a high-profile black-tie event to sustain and expand programming.

As demonstrated by Candi and Sarah, the bane of Black autism mothers' existence was not limited to White-dominated autism cultural spaces. Mothers maintained connections to Black cultural spaces, including sororities, community events, and churches. Black cultural connections were important to BAMs because they valued and needed to be in social and spiritual community with other Black women and families. Participating mothers prioritized their sons' needs but also resisted allowing autism to take full control of their lives. Their sons' autism and associated behaviors, however, led Black autism mothers to find Black cultural spaces where autism was recognized and understood; they sought out Black cultural spaces where their sons would be treated well and accepted.

Autism in Black Churches

Black autism mothers may not have actively sought participation in autism cultural spaces, but most actively engaged in Black church communities as members, leaders, and even pastors' wives. Participants cited church as a source of social, political, and spiritual activities. While most had positive interactions with church members, a few mothers described instances of members' hurtful behaviors toward them and their sons. Their negative experiences are echoed in research on Black churches and disabilities, with some members demonstrating rigidity to inclusiveness of autistic children in church activities. A lack of autism knowledge and awareness caused some participants to feel unwelcome in church settings (King, 1998; Rose, 1997).

From the time Michelle received Sam's autism diagnosis, she committed to creating a community for him where he would be immersed in Black culture. Michelle feared that social isolation was not only unhealthy for Sam but also for herself, because she "was a community person." She remained undaunted and determined to expose Sam to Black cultural events in a variety of settings. Michelle explained her reasoning: "I wasn't shutting him away; we were going to be out in the community. I never shied away and said we can't go. We may not stay the entire time, or we may need a little support, but I'm going to give it a try. That was always my stance that we could do it. We were going to try." An active young man, Sam loves to jump, clap his hands, and run, activities that in spaces like church raise alarms. Black women's long-standing struggle for recognition of their personhood left Michelle undeterred and unbothered by stares and disapproving looks in response to Sam's behaviors. She drew upon emancipatory ideas by saying, "We come from a legacy of people who are survivors, people who persevere. We are not thin skinned when it comes to having people stare and be the only ones. That same thing is what I use when I'm dealing with something related to Sam. I don't let anybody else define who I am, what my limitations are, or capabilities and the same is true for my son." While Sam's behaviors caused people to stare at times, Michelle confidently moved through public spaces undeterred by glares or astonished expressions. I should note that we attended the same church and I watched how Michelle maneuvered with Sam in public spaces. People were initially uncomfortable with Sam's sudden jumping or rocking. She held his hand, gently telling him to settle down, or ignored the behaviors in the moment. Eventually, church members became comfortable with Sam, and a few even supervised him during service while Michelle engaged in other activities. She educated members about autism and the church loved and accepted mother and son. Michelle's presence was a turning point, as other families with children on the autism spectrum joined the congregation.

Despite being married to a pastor, Donelle's position as "First Lady" did not insulate her family from church members' hurtful comments in response to her son Bear's autism-related behaviors. She described how years ago Black churches had limited understanding and patience with special needs individuals or those who present as "different." She said, "The church is not prepared for those who are different," noting that "only in the last 10 years" has she seen a slight shift in attitudes toward Bear. Perhaps congregants had grown used to Bear, but Donelle noticed that congregants now demonstrate awareness of autism and exercise patience when dealing with him. Donelle was not lulled into believing that the passage of time changed church members' feelings about Bear as she bluntly shared, "People don't love him. He talks incessantly, he is loud and doesn't recognize how loud he is."

In the years immediately following Pappas's autism diagnosis, Candi described longing for a church where Pappas would be loved, nurtured, and accepted. She wanted a Black church that would function as an extended family with church school offerings for Pappas. This was not the case for her family, as she recalled being dismissed from two church congregations before joining a congregation that embraced her family. According to Candi, "We done got thrown out of two churches. Don't get it twisted." According to Candi, Pappas was unwelcomed in the first church because his autism-related behaviors were misunderstood. In response to several instances where church members expressed discomfort with Pappas, Candi confronted members who spoke despairingly of him. Candi recalled how she "went off" one Sunday, telling a few select church members, "I'm tired, I'm tired. I'm tired. Y'all gonna stop speaking that way, acting that way, and y'all supposed to be representing Christians. I went off on the deacon's wife and told the financial lady that I was waiting for her in the parking lot. I went off." In traditional Black churches, deacons, their wives, and church officers hold symbolic, financial, and cultural power in congregations and are recognized as leaders. By virtue of confronting powerful church members, Candi received dismissal letters following the incident, with church leaders reportedly making no efforts at conflict resolution. The receipt of three letters added insult to injury with Candi saying, "I was more mad that they wrote a letter for Pappas too. [I felt like], how dare you put my baby's name on the letter. They gave us three separate letters. They wrote a letter for me, a letter for my husband, and a letter for Pappas."

Following that experience, Candi continued the search for a church home. She joined another church, where she participated in the youth ministry, in order to ensure Pappas's safety and respectful treatment. After 3 years, she became disenchanted with the second church for the same reason as the first—Pappas's treatment and the stifling ignorance of church members toward autism. Despite her service as a Sunday school teacher, she shared how members became hesitant to leave their children in Pappas's class because they did not understand his behaviors. She shared that one Sunday, she had enough of the mistreatment and confronted a woman who deemed Pappas's behaviors as harmful for the safety of other children. Candi elaborated, saying, "One day, a lady actually looked at him and said, 'Oh, ain't nobody safe at Sunday school.' I said, 'Lord hold me, you better hold me, because I'm 'bout to get her.'" Candi recalled responding to the lady by saying, "You do know autism is not contagious and my son is bound to catch the flu from your child before your child catches autism from him. You do know that? Because people were acting like they couldn't be around him." Candi then humorously shared how her best friend, who also attended the church, begged her to let the offense go. She said, "Oh, I'm waiting for you in the parking lot. My girlfriend begged me, please go home. I was like, 'Nope, I'm not going home. She gotta watch her mouth. Not my baby. You can say whatever you want to me, but you going to leave my baby alone.'" After some time, Candi found a church where Pappas is treated with respect, although she still fights efforts to exclude him.

Emphasizing that all children are God's children, Candi fought for Pappas's inclusion in Easter plays and out-of-town Sunday school trips. The church welcomed the creation of a special needs class, taught by Candi, because other Sunday school teachers did not want to work with them. On church trips, special needs children that were formerly excluded now share a room with her and Pappas and sit with them on the bus. She reminds the other teachers that Jesus walked among the deaf, mute, and maimed, saying, "[I tell them] 'did you read the part where Jesus said bring the little children unto me? He didn't specify bring the honor students and the non–special needs kids.'" Candi was not afraid to directly address those perpetrating unkindness upon Pappas and challenging those in power to change themselves and their organizations.

Black autism mothers' experiences in churches speaks to the overarching need for Black autism cultural spaces. Participants were asked to share ideas of what a Black autism cultural space would look, sound, and feel like, as BAMs were encouraged to engage their senses when thinking about the possibilities of such a space. Marley, who began this section describing her desire for an autism community, delighted in thinking about an unapologetically Black space. She bravely conceptualized a "healing autism house" geared toward providing culturally competent autism services for Black families.

> It would be in the city. It would be somewhere where we can all get together, whether you have a car or don't. Our children are getting together, they are creating relationships, but it's holistic. It's not anything forced . . . everyone's invited but

you need to be able to contribute something . . . a healing home, where we can get together, you know like in the south where Big Momma has cooked something, you can get a meal. There is a person of color that can give some therapy session, because it's different. It's different from me talking to you than I would Sally. It's just different. Then in the backyard kids are playing safely.

Marley elaborated on the "healing autism house," noting that the space would be a safe, healing space for BAMs with attention to therapy, sessions on self-care, and management of caregiver stress. She further elaborated upon her dream Black autism space by adding: "Having this autistic healing house to where you leave better than you came, you leave with resources. We need to not just talk about the autism part, but that mental health part of mothers and taking care of ourselves, and the mental illness part and the trauma that our kid will face and how do we deal with that in the community . . ." The autism healing house, participants' nonprofit missions, and BAMs' descriptions of ideal church environments collectively represent soft places for BAMs to land—Black autism cultural spaces where they can be vulnerable, seek assistance with no judgment, and interact with other families who have shared experiences. Conceptualizations of ideal Black autism spaces reflect culturally responsive care that taps into Black autism mothers' perspectives, needs, and recognizes their presence in autism. In the next section, Black autism mothers further illuminate these themes with a focus on the need for culturally responsive autism care and services.

BAMs Offer Advice on Culturally Responsive Autism Care and Services

Access to quality autism services is of central importance to autism families across the racial and class spectrum. Black families across income levels experience disparities in diagnosis, care, and treatment for Black autistic children (Burkett et al., 2015; Clark, 2014; Cuccaro et al., 2007; Mandell et al., 2009). Black children are diagnosed at later ages than their White peers and misdiagnosed with non-autism conditions, further prolonging the diagnosis timeline spanning 3 years (Constantino et al., 2020; Stahmer et al., 2019). Research examining disparities in outcomes for Black autistic children points to anti-Black racism and bias held by health care professionals, coupled with limited access to care as discriminatory drivers, even when controlling for income and education levels (Burkett et al., 2015; Constantino et al., 2020; Straiton & Sridhar, 2022).

As Black autism mothers in this study and elsewhere attest to, service delivery of clinicians and service providers centers the experiences of White middle-class families, leaving Black families without culturally competent health care and services. Betancourt et al. (2003) define culturally competent health care as:

> [Care that] acknowledges and incorporates—at all levels—the importance of culture, assessment of cross-cultural relations, vigilance toward the dynamics that result from cultural differences, expansion of cultural knowledge, and adaptation of services to meet culturally unique needs. A culturally competent system is also built on an awareness of the integration and interaction of health beliefs and behaviors, disease prevalence and incidence, and treatment outcomes for different patient populations . . . the field of cultural competence has recognized the inherent challenges in attempting to disentangle social factors (socioeconomic factors, supports/stressors, environmental hazards) from cultural factors vis-à-vis their influence on the individual patient. (p. 204)

Providers act out racial and culturally held beliefs that subsequently translate into diagnosis, care, and treatment decisions.

The need for cultural competence and the continued centering of White autism families complicated BAMs' self-described relationships with providers, as they wanted providers who understood Black family dynamics. Moreover, BAMs wanted professionals to respectfully approach them free of deficit-based assumptions of their sons and families. By "talking back," that is, asserting themselves with clinical and service providers, BAMs resisted negative perceptions of Black children and families. They approached clinicians and service providers expecting to confront negative perceptions with counternarratives of strength and resilience about their sons and families. BAMs wanted providers to bring a holistic understanding of Black patients and families through the lens of culturally responsive care that acknowledges how sociopolitical, economic, and cultural forces frame Black life in America. Within the confines of this study, Black autism mothers "talk back" to providers, collectively sharing concerns and advice on how providers can learn and exercise culturally responsive care for Black autism families.

Educational scholars Geneva Gay (2010) and Gloria Ladson-Billings (1995) developed the field of culturally responsive/relevant pedagogy, which I am liberally applying here to better flesh out BAMs' advice on improved culturally responsive services. As a teaching practice, culturally responsive teaching encompasses three key principles: sociopolitical consciousness, cultural competence, and academic achievement. Acknowledgment of societal injustices that impact students, families, communities, and schools is essential for culturally responsive educators. For purposes of this study, sociopolitical consciousness means clinicians and service care providers must acknowledge that race, class, and gender impact health and service outcomes for Blacks.

The concept of cultural competence requires that providers understand how their services recognize the humanness of Black families, that is, providing clinical spaces where Black families can unapologetically be themselves in judgment-free spaces (Carr & Lord, 2012; Delgado Rivera & Rogers-Atkinson, 1997; Leininger, 1991; Leininger & McFarland, 2006). While academic achievement does not directly apply to this study, the concept translates to this study as it encompasses practices of developing and holding high expectations for Black families and individual clients, as opposed to stereotypical deficit notions of Black family structures. Academic achievement, or high expectations, in this sense, refers to professionals maintaining high standards of care for Black autism families. High expectations further translate into maintaining an openness to parental knowledge, respecting parents' knowledge of their children, and integrating parental knowledge into treatment. These interpretations of culturally responsive teaching align with social work and human services literature that emphasizes that an awareness of White privilege and race-based systemic oppression facilitates practitioners' ability to integrate such awareness into practices (Davis & Gentlewarrior, 2015; Priester et al., 2017). In doing so, White practitioners demonstrate sociopolitical consciousness and cultural competence, thereby reducing the imposition of racial stereotypes and facilitating the establishment of client–practitioner relationships (Priester et al., 2017).

Sociopolitical Consciousness

With regard to practitioners' sociopolitical consciousness, participating Black mothers wanted service providers to recognize the ways in which race and class impact their families. They wanted providers to understand that seeking services presented a host of challenges that are not necessarily visible when providers interact with Black families at appointments. Thelma spoke on the challenges of receiving quality services as a Black mother who at times faced dire financial challenges. She described her struggle to receive services for Elijah and Solomon: "In order to get good quality services, you have to become colorless. We become colorless and more until your son becomes the young Black man who is over 6 feet tall." Thelma illustrated her "becoming colorless" strategy during our interview by shifting into a higher vocal register and purposefully over enunciating her words as she detailed the obstacles faced just to receive services. Her comments further allude to BAMs' awareness and responses to racial differentiation in autism service delivery.

When specifically speaking of medical providers, Black autism mothers interacted almost exclusively with White providers whom they believed failed to fully comprehend why Black families approach medical providers with apprehension and distrust. Washington (2006) recounts the tenuous relationship between Black communities and large medical facilities due to a history of medical experimentation on Blacks, most notably the Tuskegee Syphilis Study and the story of Henrietta Lacks (Jones & Mandell, 2020; Nickerson et al., 1994). Study participants like Donelle were aware not only of the troubling history of medical experimentation on Blacks but also disparities in health outcomes for Black people. The political mindsets of BAMs made them leery of doctors' recommendations, especially given their concerns of being invisibilized, unheard, and dismissed. BAMs were willing to work with medical professionals but wanted their experiential knowledge respected and considered in treatment plans. For example, Donelle recounted being thrown out of a neuropsychologist's office early in 31-year-old Bear's autism journey because she disagreed with the doctor's stance on using medicine to address Bear's behaviors. Based on her experiences, she cautioned medical providers to consider other strategies and advised providers, "Don't be so quick to prescribe meds." Given the troubling historical and contemporary context of Black health outcomes, Donelle was skeptical about medications as the lone course of action.

Sociopolitical consciousness does not entail providers having aligned political views with Black autism families. The concept should also not be reduced to shared political party affiliation either. Instead, Black autism mothers wanted medical professionals to understand that treatment strategies are influenced by social factors including race, geographic access, and economic status. Karla wanted medical practitioners to directly address race with families to foster better understandings of familial contexts outside the confines of clinical spaces. Practitioners that demonstrated an awareness of race, she believed, could then address root causes of Black family stress and trauma that may impact patients. She shared the following suggestion for autism professionals to inform culturally responsive approaches:

> I would say, asking questions; questions like what's important to a person's family. Asking how they communicate, how they interact with each other. What sorts of things do they do with each other? But also ask them the question as far as, how are they responding, and their families and their children responding to what's going on in our society? As far as race, or what their children know? And what do our children know? And how is the family going to respond? Just asking about that.

As suggested by Karla, critical questions are a means of learning from Black families but also establishing relationships with Black autism families. Clinicians can use critical questions to learn firsthand about health and service disparities impacting Black autism families. Critical questions also serve to humanize Black families while expanding conceptualizations of autism families beyond White familial norms: not all autism mothers are White.

Cultural Competence

Study participants pointed to cultural competence as an important cornerstone in working with Black families seeking autism care. BAMs' references to cultural competence were multidimensional and encompassed: understanding Black familial values, beliefs, and childrearing approaches; the need for Black health care and autism service providers; and the equity work within organizations serving autism families. Black family values included faith, as BAMS leaned not on their worldly understanding of autism but relied heavily on spiritual guidance when making critical decisions for their sons. For example, Ginger's faith undergirds how she makes meaning of mothering two sons on the autism spectrum. A medical professional or service provider working with Ginger's family must understand that faith is a stabilizing force in her life that enables her to care for her two adult sons with autism. She advised providers to "treat Black families and kids with respect, honor, and dignity as their own." Ginger elaborated on her steadfast faith by adding, "I am not afraid to tell [service providers] that the God of the universe, He can make a tree. He can rewire the brain, chromosomes. He has an arsenal in heaven. I am foolish enough to believe that this God can do anything." She preferred medical providers whose cultural competence extended into a faith walk, where they could balance science with faith.

Participants collectively pointed to the presence of Black medical professionals and service providers as a critical component to providing culturally competent services. For example, vestiges of deep-seated historical racial trauma continually haunt Black family life and health outcomes. Marley drew upon DeGruy's (2005) concept of post-traumatic slave syndrome to frame her comments about how historical trauma still impacts Black families in ways that, although hard to articulate, could be innately understood by Black health care providers. She added:

> [It] doesn't just start with my child having autism. This is some stuff as family as Black and brown family. We've got to deal with some trauma that has been leaving some baggage that we have been carrying since slavery. We don't even know that we carry. You as a White person won't get that. Sometimes I can't put words to it. But I believe that a Black practitioner will say, "I got it, I got you." They can pick up where I can't. They have words. They can help me articulate it better. They also know my tears that I would cry are not just tears of why, it's not a "Why me?" It's so much more.

Black autism mothers may want to connect with autism providers on a relational level; however, such efforts are thwarted by providers' lack of cultural competency, which requires mutual openness, respect, and shared cultural knowledge. Given the lack of cultural competence of medical professionals and service providers, Black mothers felt the weight of explaining and defending how Black families think, behave, and function fell on them like a burden they were uninterested in carrying. Mothers believed that cultural competence facilitated delivery of appropriate medical care that fits the needs of Black families. Care without cultural competence essentially meant that Black autism families were receiving treatment normed on White middle-class families and treatment that failed to account for sociohistorical contexts that impact daily Black life.

The presence of Black practitioners would provide a sense of relief—a reprieve from constantly explaining belief systems, values, and culturally informed parenting practices. Black practitioners can bring subjugated knowledge to bear on autism practices, which is the experiential knowledge of Black family dynamics, laying the foundation for autism care enhanced by experiential knowledge of Black life in America. Black autism professionals, like doctors, psychologists, and social workers who exercise cultural competence, provide Black autism mothers much-needed and rare spaces of cultural understanding. While a few participants noted how the onus of cultural competence, in many ways, tends to fall on people of color, they considered Black clinicians better prepared to provide culturally competent services.

Organizations serving autism families must have greater accountability for ensuring culturally competent services and work in partnership with Black families (Pearson & Meadan, 2021). Black autism mothers in this study believed that Black representation is needed around leadership tables where key decisions are made. For example, years spent as a nonprofit CEO informed Indigo's insistence that greater Black representation around the decision-making table directly impacts cultural competence within health care and autism service organizations. Indigo was uniquely positioned to provide insights on how agencies and funders make decisions that impact Black families absent of Black representation. Indigo shared a recent opportunity to serve on a statewide advisory board for individuals with disabilities. She explained that she jumped at the opportunity because she could bring her experiences to the table: a Black autism mother and nonprofit CEO. Participation in the statewide committee reified her belief that representation matters, as she saw firsthand how funding does not always get distributed to Black urban communities. She recalled the experience:

> So, I put it out there to make sure that they knew that's what I meant, because the email, and the call for the advisory board did speak to communities of color, but that doesn't mean that we're around the table making the decision, right? Particularly

about who you fund. So, when money is distributed, there's always the big organizations that always gets the money, because they provide service, but there is a gap in their service to communities of color, with a cultural competency foundation to it.

When asked to elaborate upon what the proverbial "table" should look like, Indigo again spoke from her professional and personal experiences as a Black autism mother. The "table" must have racial and socioeconomic representation to better reflect the interests of communities of color. Indigo explained:

> First of all, making sure that conversation and systems that are set up, are set up uniformly, and not making assumptions about people, whatever their zip code is. I also would think that the reality of the matter is that many communities of color that have kids dealing with trauma are in high poverty communities. So, the allocation and the resources necessary for agencies providing service to those communities, it can't be proportionally uniform. It would involve people from communities of color in the decision making, when funding allocations are made.

Indigo's comments further demonstrate that Black autism mothers understand how Black representation around the decision-making table will impact the quality and delivery of autism services.

High Expectations for Clinicians and Autism Researchers

Across participants in this study, high expectations were interpreted as service providers eliminating long-standing practices of stereotyping Black families upon sight, thereby limiting treatment options and life outcomes. For example, Gourdine et al. (2011) highlighted the case of a professional Black couple, parents of a child with autism, who were subjected to judgmental and harsh comments during the evaluation process. The psychologist made judgments based upon the family's race and perceived socioeconomic status, only to learn that the parents were highly educated, and not uneducated as was originally presumed. This incident demonstrates the ways in which provider perceptions, or misperceptions, can shape service delivery, as the family involved received a poor prognosis about their son's life outcomes—a prognosis delivered with judgment of the family as unenlightened. BAMs wanted professionals to deliver care consistent to that received by White middle- to upper middle-class families. Straiton and Sridhar (2022) call upon autism clinicians to listen to Black autistic people and their families' opinions about services. The researchers also argue that clinicians must resolve service hurdles that Black families encounter when navigating service pathways. Thus, acknowledging that Black families' social and economic positionality elongates service timelines; anti-Black racism has implications for immediate and long-term prognosis and service access.

While participants focused primarily on clinical and autism services, autism disparities also point to the underrepresentation of Black families in autism research. More recent research attests to the need for Black family participation in autism research to improve health outcomes and racial health disparities (Jones & Mandell, 2020; Shaia et al., 2020). The reasons for limited Black participation in autism studies, including genome research, vary, but experts cite transportation, work schedules of working-class families, and long-standing distrust of research (Jones & Mandell, 2020; Yee, 2016). With regard to genome research specifically, Yee's (2016) *Atlantic* monthly article on racial bias in autism research noted that Black family structures may also contribute to restricting Black families from genome research:

> Household structure is one barrier to participating in genetic studies. Most typically require DNA samples from parents and siblings of a child with autism, but many black children don't live in two-parent households with siblings who share the same parents. (In 2013, 67 percent of black children in the U.S. lived in a single-parent household, compared with 25 percent of white children.) In 2008, blacks accounted for only 2.3 percent of the participants in the Autism Genetic Resource Exchange gene bank. (p. 4)

Arguably, the reasons for Black underrepresentation in autism research must be taken with some caution. Rationales related to access, distrust, and other constraints are important, yet they simultaneously build upon social and medical pathologies of Black families. Black family structures do not necessarily mean that nonresidential Black fathers are not accessible or uninvolved in their children's lives (Cabrera et al., 2008; King et al., 2004). The rationale also fails to consider the often-overlooked complexities of class diversity that exist within Black communities and, specifically, Black autism families. As a reminder, all 14 ($N = 14$) BAMs participating in this study are college educated and hold professional positions. Yet only two of 14 participants (14%) had ever been involved in autism studies, even though all participants lived in regions with autism research centers and large clinical research settings. And most participants were married, in partnerships, or had contact with their children's fathers.

The onus of limited research participation of Black families should not be placed on families, but researchers must look closely at intentionality of exclusion due to racial and class bias. For example, Michelle spoke passionately about how autism research views Black families through a deficit lens not to the detriment of Black autistic individuals but to autism research. She was critical of researchers reifying racial bias through intentional exclusion of Blacks and their inscription of negative stereotypes on Black autistic children. Michelle said,

> Systems must stop labeling Black kids. They pigeonhole them, limit their expectations, and define what their path is going to be. When they do that, it's done through a lens skewed by racism, low expectations, bias, and perspectives that says this person isn't entitled to a certain humanity. That stuff needs to be called out! If we move in the world thinking we live in a colorless and raceless society, we're being naïve. Decisions are made all the time that impact people across racial lines.

Autism research is not free of racial bias, as researchers bring personal beliefs that then translate into systemic labeling of Black kids.

Systemic inactions and stereotyping can directly impact improved access to medical breakthroughs for Black autism families. Michelle believed that access to new remedies, such as that afforded through research studies, is limited to White families with money and social capital in autism circles. She stated:

> Everyone should have options. It's not right that only certain groups of people even know about this information and that there's loads of other people who are experiencing these same issues, that have these same challenges, that could benefit from

these services, but don't even know it exists. Treat our kids as your kids. The same things you want for your child is the same thing I want. As we move through this world, the same opportunities, access, and experiences that they have are not the same experiences that we have. Race does play a factor, gender plays a factor, and class plays a factor.

Although most participants described apprehension of medicines, opportunities to participate in research studies or innovative treatments should not be limited to White families. Autism researchers and clinicians must take responsibility for the preponderance of Whiteness in autism research and work to remedy racial and class bias (Broder-Fingert et al., 2020; Shaia et al., 2020; Stahmer et al., 2019; Steinbrenner et al., 2022). Whether they choose to acknowledge their role, autism researchers and clinicians bear responsibility in the continued practice of centering Whiteness in autism assessments, treatments, and services that collectively contribute to public perceptions of autism as a White condition.

High Expectations for Service Care Coordinators and Agencies

Service coordinators who are responsible for shepherding families to community-based, state, and federal services bore the brunt of BAMs' criticisms, as mothers held high standards and expectations of service providers. Social workers and other human services professionals play an important role for autism families; these professionals identify gaps in care, identify available services, and navigate complex systems to help families access childcare, therapeutic treatments, and other community-based services. Agencies also provide autism families a lifeline to respite services and autism families rely upon agency services and value consistent relationships with service providers.

Participants were alarmed by instability in care because they depended on consistent services that enabled them to work full-time and maintain a modicum of much-needed self-care. For example, Kendra depended upon a community-based agency to provide her twin boys with after-school care and full-time summer programming. She was pleased with the agency staff and believed they genuinely care about her sons. Shortly before our interview, news broke that the agency was suddenly closing. Reports were initially vague, but it was later revealed that the agency leadership mismanaged federal funds. Kendra was among a few hundred parents left scrambling for services. The agency said they would help families locate comparable care, but many families were left juggling schedules and relying upon family networks for care. While Kendra was able to locate services for the boys, transitions for children on the spectrum can prove challenging and the closure upset her twins, who had grown accustomed to the agency staff.

Service disruptions were a common theme among Black autism mothers, many of whom were frustrated with high turnover among service care providers. BAMs were dissatisfied by service disruptions due to service coordinators leaving agencies, sometimes with little notice to families. The aftermath of service coordinators' departures required Black autism mothers to start over in building relationships with coordinators. Relationships were critical because service care advocacy is contingent upon how well the coordinator knows the client and the family. They must then work in the interest of individuals and families based on their articulated needs. Personnel changes necessitated BAMs telling their autism narratives, completing additional paperwork, and as some mothers articulated, starting over from square one. Thus, the revolving door of care coordinators placed BAMs and their sons in a vulnerable position, as they relied upon services. Staffing changes also resulted in lingering feelings of mistrust toward agencies.

To be fair, high turnover among human service professionals is not uncommon and due to a variety of factors. Research points to fatigue, toxic organizations, emotional labor, low pay, and general job dissatisfaction as sources of professional burnout (Ducharme et al., 2007). Lisa felt empathy for care coordinators and recognized the high stress–low pay nature of their positions. She acknowledged that low pay was a primary motivator for educated individuals to leave positions within the human service field, and she shared her frustration by commenting:

> I don't know, maybe we need to talk about having people paid more fairly for doing these kinds of human service jobs that are so important, so there can be some consistency and you don't have to have people working two or three jobs. A guy who was our service coordinator probably got a degree in psychology, and was like, and probably even maybe got it from private schools. He got a job doing Medicaid service coordination. It wasn't enough, $20,000 or $30,000, so maybe he has another job. I get it.

At the time of our interview, Lisa was faced with finding yet another service coordinator, as John's coordinator left the agency and did not provide advance notice to Lisa.

Consequently, Lisa's family was left in need of respite and after-school care for John. While she recognized that low pay may have factored into her coordinator's departure, she was equally perturbed by what she perceived as a lack of respect on his part, as she did not have time to prepare for changes. She believed he failed in his duties and stated: "You still have a job to do, and he completely let me down. He completely let my kid down. Then you don't even, you don't even own up to it. You don't apologize. You just don't return my call at all. Just, I guess, hoping I'll go away. I'm just so angry about that! Now I gotta go through this whole process all again!" The service provider left her with limited options, negated her trust, and demonstrated a lack of respect for John.

Beverly had also reached the point of frustration with her family's care coordinator, as she too was dealing with the loss of a coordinator due to turnover. The staffing inconsistencies caused her to rethink her approach to working with care coordinators, as she determined to use a more formal cautious approach moving forward. "I don't want them even in my house. Every time you turn around, every 6 months they're quitting and we're getting a new one and a new one and a new one. So, I'm not bringing all them people up in my house. I'm telling you right now. Meet me at McDonald's. This can be my meeting point. I'm definitely done!" The decision to meet at the local McDonald's created a more formal approach to dealing with care coordinators, as opposed to her previous approach of inviting them into the intimacy of her home. The act of opening her home speaks to the emotional energy needed to engage with care coordinators, as mothers shared their time, space, and autism narratives. The perceived lack of respect resulted in Beverly considering another agency to coordinate 16-year-old Marvelous's case. "I'm about to look for somebody else. They don't do nothing. They are ripping off Medicaid. They don't do nothing. In order for me to get other things, I have to have them, but they don't do jack. I just got a letter from them saying if they don't hear from me, they're going to close my case. So, I only keep them open so I can get services but I'm about to tell them, I'm about to leave them." The constant staff turnover also led her to reassess what services the agency provided, as Beverly faced a service conundrum—she needed the agency to get services, but she did not trust the agency to act in her family's best interest.

Chapter Summary

At the intersection of race, class, gender, and autism, Black mothers encountered images of autism mothering that invisibilized them while centralizing the experiences of White middle-class mothers. A few attempted to participate in autism cultural spaces, that is, formalized spaces of autism services, programming, and social media focused on autism. Prevailing images of autism families serve to deter Black family participation in autism culture, as exclusionary messages of who is an autism mother and how autism mothers function as warriors prevail. Instead, Black autism mothers approached autism spaces with apprehension while most chose not to engage in spaces dominated by White autism mothers. The need to create autism spaces that addressed access to autism services in communities of color motivated two study participants to create their own nonprofit organizations.

Black autism mothering encompassed political advocacy leveraged by Black women to ensure positive life outcomes for their sons. Participating mothers attempted to hold human service agencies and care coordinators accountable for their actions and delivery of services (Carr & Lord, 2012; Delgado Rivera & Rogers-Atkinson, 1997; Leininger, 1991; Leininger & McFarland, 2006). Black mothers "spoke back to" clinical and service providers with experiential knowledge of why and how culturally responsive services are needed. The advocacy of Black autism mothers for acceptance and respect also extended to Black churches, with a few mothers describing how they pushed church members to move past ignorance to acceptance. Their experiences attest to the need for inclusive representations of Black families in representations of autism.

Chapter 7

BAMs and the Future

By the age of 12, Caleb's behaviors began to ratchet exponentially related to anxiety, obsessive-compulsive disorder, tics, and ADHD: all comorbid conditions to his autism. The addition of hormonal shifts also contributed to the unpredictability of his behaviors. His perseverations intensified to the point of lasting for hours. He would literally get stuck on saying, "I'm sorry." What started in the evening over a small directive, such as picking up socks, or using a napkin, would literally last into the early morning, or follow him onto the school bus.

"Caleb, come in here and clear your plate."

"I'm sorry. I'm sorry." This phrase would be repeated at least 10 to 12 times.

"Okay, I hear you. I need you to stop, get unstuck. How can I help you?"

"Just say you accept my apology."

"Caleb, I accept your apology. You're okay. It's cool."

"It's cool?"

"Yes, it's cool. You're fine. You're a good person. You just need to clean up your mess."

"Okay, thank you for accepting my apology."

"You're welcome."

"Can you say it again?"

The conversation would continue to spiral with him repeating his apologetic plea. If the incident took place in public, I quickly had to gather our belongings and leave, out of fear that bystanders would call the police, mistaking his perseverative fit as a response to abuse on my part. Or, if the perseverative fit took place while in the confines of our home, it was not out of the ordinary for the fixations to result in physical aggression. Subsequently, each fit yielded damage to various items and corners of the house. The cute Mickey Mouse television that found its way into the backyard, beaten in a fit of anger and anxiety. The bedroom furniture with wooden trim torn in response to being told, "No," the word that served as a trigger.

Meds were not my first choice to assist with managing Caleb's behaviors. My views shifted, however, as his in-school behaviors intensified. There were calls from school with concerns regarding intensified behaviors, including running out of class, screaming in the hallways, and hitting classmates with his belt. I began to view meds as a means of helping him function better across the day. I did my reading on various drugs being used with children with ASD and felt informed. He needed a combination of medicines to address anxiety, aggression, OCD, and tics.

We then connected with an adolescent psychiatric unit of the local university and began a combination of behavioral therapy and medicine to address his needs. Over time, the psychiatric appointments intended to manage his meds were increasingly challenging to book due primarily to limited adolescent psychiatric services in the area. The limited services were further punctuated by the crowded clinic lobby with little in the way of creature comforts, including waiting room seating, for the disgruntled parents and caregivers.

After a period of trial and error with several medicines, my husband and I kept hoping for a medicine combination that could keep up with Caleb's shifting hormones. His provider was a resident from the medical school, who, shortly after Caleb had a major medicine change, completed his residency and relocated. We were left without psychiatric assistance, but also, most notably, refills of powerful meds. The office refused to assign another provider.

Our family support system included me, my husband, parents, godmother, niece, and sister. My mother even retired from work to assist with his care. We patched together a caregiving schedule aligned with his school and my work schedule. Caleb became increasingly aggressive with members of our safety net. He was a sweet boy; however, he grew agitated and often expressed his frustration through aggression. One day while at work I received a call that he became aggressive with my mother. My parents had no options but to take him to the emergency room for a psychiatric evaluation.

In the weeks immediately following his hospitalization, we were forced to homeschool him as his school recommended he not return in such a fragile state. The district then had to coordinate efforts to locate an out-of-district therapeutic day treatment program. To further confound matters, incidents of elopement increased, resulting in calls to the police to help locate him. We were exhausted and depressed. Finally, we collectively concluded that we were not enough. He needed more than our collective efforts at safety, compassion, and love could provide. I am Caleb's mom, and, in this moment, I realize he needs more support. We were not enough.

∼

The pathway of parenting a son with autism is never smooth or easy; to the contrary, it is filled with critical questions and important developmental junctures. As discussed across the book, Black autism mothers must make decisions related to their children's diagnosis, schooling, autism care, and services. One of the weightiest decisions for Black autism mothers relates to long-term care and decision-making. The question of "what's next" is deceivingly oversimplified, as BAMs must consider what the future holds for their sons at the intersection of race, class, gender, and autism. While most participants made decisions in collaboration with spouses and family members, the emotional weight fell heavily upon mothers who balanced realities of their son's current needs with considerations of what the future might hold.

This chapter examines Black autism mothers' hopes for the future, as they describe hopes for their sons' lives. Participating mothers were aware of the challenges they faced in securing long-term care and living arrangements, while simultaneously considering their own life spans. The research literature on life outcomes for Black adults with autism paints a bleak picture of service disconnection, unemployment, and poor health outcomes. Despite these outcomes, Black autism mothers were collectively optimistic and instead chose to channel their efforts on ensuring their sons were Black men of character; they placed energy on ensuring their sons were "good Black men."

The Dearth of Adult Autism Services

Black autism mothers throughout this study attest to the challenges of securing a range of autism services in K–12 schooling. In a perfect world, K–12 schooling environments provide a service ecosystem driven by annual IEP goals. Students with autism can receive daily or weekly delivery of services, including speech and occupational therapy, social skills groups, vocational training, mental health counseling, and other services required by law. Schools also play a role in transitioning students with autism into adulthood as federal law requires transition planning beginning at age 16. Under ideal circumstances, families participate in transition planning, partnering with school and district staff to determine the next steps for their children. Federal mandates, however, do not require sustained autism services into adulthood (Eilenberg et al., 2019), creating what autism experts liken to "falling off a cliff" (Roux et al., 2015, p. 8), leaving many families disconnected from critical services (Malone et al., 2022). Researchers also note that the needs of adults with autism intensify because they must navigate employment, independent living, and postsecondary options (Eilenberg et al., 2019; Shattuck et al., 2012). Additionally, the presence of comorbid conditions including depression, anxiety, ADHD, OCD, and other maladaptive behaviors can also intensify during the transition to adulthood without sustained mental health services (Eilenberg et al., 2019; Hendricks & Wehman, 2009; Roux et al., 2015; Taylor & Seltzer, 2011).

Postsecondary options depend on a variety of factors, including parental income, availability of training, social supports, and individual needs. Some adults on the autism spectrum are able to locate and maintain employment with the assistance of job coaches. Donelle's adult son Bear worked at a fast-food restaurant and received job coaching support. His paid position, however, was not full-time and was low wage. In addition to job coaching, postsecondary opportunities for autistic adults also include competitive employment, day programming incorporating community service, unstructured activities, and college (including specialized autism programs that provide social and academic supports) (Taylor & Seltzer, 2011, p. 6). For example, Ginger's adult sons Cat Man and Music Man participated in a day support program every day. They received transportation from home and participated in community volunteer projects such as recycling, paper shredding, and Meals on Wheels. The sheltered program included individuals from across the autism spectrum with varying communication skills.

According to Ennis-Cole et al. (2013) however, community-based employment opportunities are limited for young adults and adults with autism. Lisa worried not only about available opportunities but about what jobs were a match for her son. John, 16, is minimally verbal and struggled with social connections. Undeterred, she contemplated if John's food obsession could translate into a job opportunity and drive his interest toward baking. As we discussed the possibility of sheltered community employment opportunities, Lisa worried about John's hygiene and thought better of jobs involving food service and preparation. She pondered his future possibilities, saying, "Well could he work at a bakery, and dump ingredients into a pot? But then there's also things you have to do. You have to be clean and you have to wash your hands. There's a lot of other things that go along with having a job than just knowing the things that go into a pot." Since John was 16 years old, Lisa was on the cusp of working with school staff to develop a transition plan for him.

Across autism quality-of-life indicators White adults with autism from high-income families have better employment outcomes and higher rates of independent living (Roux et al., 2015; Taylor & Seltzer, 2011). Wealthy White families leverage social capital and income to create jobs and independent living opportunities for their children. Black adults on the autism spectrum, however, experience disparities across quality-of-life outcomes and are less likely to live independently, be employed, pursue postsecondary opportunities, and maintain autism services. The fall is even steeper for Black autistic adults, who are disconnected from autism services at rates greater than their White peers.

The next section expounds upon the connection of quality-of-life outcomes to Black autism mothers' expectations for their sons. What deserves further exploration related to quality-of-life outcomes is how Black autism mothers conceptualize and approach adult transitions (Kirby, 2016). Participating mothers grappled with what independence means for their sons at the intersection of race, class, gender, and autism. BAMs took autism into account but refused to lower expectations and, instead, established expectations based on their sons' social, physical, and communicative abilities. They were determined to raise "good" Black men and held high behavioral, social, and character expectations (Annamma et al., 2013).

Raising Successful and Good Black Men

Black mothers play a pivotal role in preparing their sons for adulthood as they instill in them kindness, respect, and a sense of responsibility (Boyd-Franklin & Franklin, 2000; Bush, 2004; Gantt & Greif, 2009; Mandara et al., 2010). Their efforts also include preparing their sons to maneuver in a society that dichotomously fears their presence yet emulates their cultural swagger (Ladson-Billings, 2011). BAMs did not discount that autism impacted their sons' lives but instead recalibrated their ideas of success in light of autism and their sons' individual strengths. Mothers conveyed conceptualizations of what it means to be a good Black man, even in the presence of autism. They were aware of employment and other long-term outcomes impacted by autism but imparted familial and cultural values in their sons. Recalibrating success, according to Kiara, entailed referring to autism in positive ways and teaching her son to tap into his unique skills. Kiara was purposeful in not using the term autism around 11-year-old Johnathan and translated autism-related skills as "superpowers" to empower him because she is cognizant of negative societal connotations of autism. She did not want his dreams and spirit crushed by misunderstandings and negative renderings of autism but created ways to empower him with a strengths-based approach. Johnathan's "superpower" changed weekly because she adjusted the "superpowers" to fit the context and help Johnathan confidently adapt to different situations in school and home. During our interview, she demonstrated her clever usage of "superpowers" by asking Johnathan to reflect on last week's "superpower." She said, "It was your big brain. You have the power to remember a lot of things, dates. He has an excellent memory. (Like if you tell him how old you are and we see you, he'll remember how old you are.) Lately your superpower has been getting 100s on spelling tests. You have a super memory." She encouraged Johnathan to read, dream, and think about the future while exposing him to various enrichment activities like theater; Kiara shared a video of him starring in his school's production of *The Little Mermaid*. As he sang and danced, Johnathan appeared comfortable on stage, engaged with peers, and happy.

Similarly, Candi was also attuned to how negative renderings of autism impacted her son's spirits and, as such, also approached autism from a strengths-based perspective. Candi believed in the power of positive affirmations and spoke positivity over Pappas daily to ensure safety, self-love, and confidence. She believed that as a young Black man with autism, Pappas should be prepared to encounter naysayers, those who discounted his alertness and intelligence and looked past his humanity (Waters, 2016). As we conversed about Pappas's daily routine, he interjected into the conversation, saying, "Show them how smart you are." Candi then explained that this was her daily mantra for Pappas, as she did not want anyone speaking negatively to him or about him. She believed in the power of a Black mother's love to guide sons and explained their connection, saying:

> The day after Dr. Schneider diagnosed him, I was sending him off to daycare. I looked at him, because that was the time where he didn't look at me, and I had to learn that, too, to stop telling him, "Look at me." Because he's looking at me peripherally. *He can see me.* He's zeroed in, so that was something I found out. Every day, I'll tell him, "You show them how smart you are. Mommy loves you. I'm proud of you." Because I knew that people were going to be like, "He can't do it." So every day, that's what I say to him before he get on that bus. Even when I'm out of town, I call him in the morning and I say it.

Candi's daily mantra was intended to provide a symbolic protective covering over him, reminding him of how he is loved.

During our interview, Pappas carefully selected his footwear and intentionally coordinated colors with his outfit. This action led Candi to further explain her secondary strategy for helping Pappas's self-esteem by attending to his appearance, as he takes great pride in clothes and sneakers, which makes him feel good about himself. She noted, "He always has money in his wallet, because I want him to have as much as what the neurotypical kids have, if possible. They go around, they got they little money, they want to buy stuff, they want to go places. I want him to have that. Those are all his sneakers and boots and stuff. He likes to look nice. They like to look nice. He likes to look nice. I want him to feel good about himself." Through his well-maintained appearance, Candi wanted to send a message to his peers and school staff that Pappas is loved, has high self-esteem, and thus is not to be targeted by those seeking to harm him. Candi believed that he would encounter adults who held low expectations for his behaviors and life outcomes. While Pappas has echolalia, his mother's words provided him with a means of advocating for himself and demonstrating agency, as he was able to repeat the words across settings when dealing with adults and peers.

As their sons advanced into adolescents, other Black autism mothers were careful to define success not by neurotypical measures of teen success but determined their own ways of establishing success for their sons. Adolescence is a time when youth earn drivers' licenses, graduate from high school, or attend high school dances. BAMs wanted sons to have similar experiences but created opportunities for sons to participate and have teenage memories. Candi held dreams of Pappas having a full life, with some semblance of a neurotypical life. Pappas is a handsome young man who has expressed an interest in girls. With her assistance, Pappas participated in his school's Valentine's Day activities, with Candi furnishing candy and flowers for a girl in whom Pappas had conveyed an interest.

Black autism mothers were careful to define success in ways that would not be dispiriting to both mother and son. For example, Sarah determined that using other people's standards of success was stressful and inappropriate; instead, she focused on developing Dwayne's strength of character, self-confidence, and independence as markers of success. Describing how and why she adjusted her conceptualizations of success for 12-year-old Dwayne, she commented,

> I had to adjust my goals for him so that he can be happy and I can be happy. So most importantly is that he become a responsible citizen, that he can socialize appropriately and have meaningful relationships, happy meaningful relationships, that he can be financially independent in society. He doesn't have to graduate from college. If he does graduate from college, that's great, as long as he has the skill. So, I'm into helping him have a skill so he can have a career. That skill could be whatever he loves, whatever's going to make him happy. I want it to be something that he can take care of himself so that he can one day have a family, a happy family. I want him to have a happy family, and a happy career, and a happy life.

According to Sarah, happiness, knowing God, and being leaders will contribute to both her sons' future well-being. And despite the presence of autism, she holds expectations that both her sons will develop into men. "I want my boys to be men, good Black men. I would prefer my sons be leaders versus followers." Black men, who, according to Sarah, are able to make decisions and lead.

"Just Because You Got Autism, You Don't Get a Pass"

BAMs recognized that at the intersection of race, class, gender, and autism, Black males must still be prepared to be active members of society. Participating mothers nurtured their sons' adaptive skills by teaching household duties and emphasizing personal hygiene. Black autism mothers did not want their sons limited by autism so they structured household duties to inculcate a strong work ethic and personal responsibility. BAMs established high standards for their sons and refused to let autism limit expectations for them, especially considering negative social expectations of Black men. Because they are raising Black men, the imperative to ensure a modicum of self-sufficiency and positive behaviors ran deep as Black mothers recognized that autism does not mitigate negative social expectations of Black men (Dow, 2016). Donelle summed the need to set high expectations and urged other BAMs: "Don't hold back on responsibilities just because of the disability. If you babify them, they are no good themselves or to anyone else."

BAMs believed that household duties prepared their sons for a world that is often unkind to Black men (Bush, 2000a; 2000b; 2004). For example, Kiara followed her pastor's advice and used neurotypical markers to set goals for Johnathan's household responsibilities. She explained:

> The best advice that I received from my pastor was treat him like a normal blank-year-old, however old he is. If he's an 8-year-old, how would you treat an 8-year-old. Treat him like a normal 8-year-old and I intend to. Now he's 11, so I treat him like a normal 11-year-old. He has chores, he has responsibilities, he makes his own breakfast in the morning; he knows how to use the microwave because when I was 11, I was halfway cooking the dinner.

As a single mother, Johnathan's ability to prepare meals and clean up after himself contributed to the household and helped lighten her load.

Lisa also spoke emphatically about holding her son John, 16, accountable for his actions. As the mother to two other children, Lisa believed it was important for all her children to have behavioral expectations. Like his siblings, John was expected to be mindful of household members and respectful to elders. For example, Lisa described how John was socialized to interact with extended family. Relationships were difficult for him to sustain but Lisa taught John to value family relationships. She said,

> I make all the kids acknowledge their grandmother, their nana, their aunt. You always must acknowledge elders. Even with him, I'm like, "Oh, come say hi to Grandma," or when we leave, "Okay, say goodbye to Grandma." Just because he's got a developmental disability doesn't mean that you get a pass on respecting the elders. You have to greet the elders hello and you have to tell the elders goodbye, so whether that's a grandmother or an auntie or whatever, there's certain standard greetings that apply to everyone. It applies to my little one, it applies to my oldest.

John's ability to communicate with elders in reciprocal conversation may be limited, but Lisa established social and behavioral expectations with his skills in mind. She would not tolerate some autism-related behaviors; she believed John understood what he was doing. In partnership with her husband, they forced John to clean up his spit and take responsibility for his actions. The couple believed that John understood right and wrong. She explained:

> If I see that he has spit on the floor or on something, I'm marching him right over to where it is by the scruff of his neck and I'm like, "You clean it up. You clean it up." I'm giving him paper towels or I'm giving him a wipe or something, and I'm like, "You have to clean this up." You know, "You've got to clean up. Clean up." Just because you're autistic doesn't mean that you can spit or you can be, or you can do these things that you're doing. I'm always saying to him, "That's not nice. Don't do that."

Lisa used the phrase "that's not nice" to emphasize socially unacceptable behaviors to John to prepare him for a society that does not easily look past Black males engaged in even the most menial acts.

BAMs stressed the importance of being honest or "keepin' it real" with their sons as they sought to prepare them for adulthood. They did not hold back when communicating with their sons because they recognized the world is not kind to Black males. BAMs communicated straightforward messages to sons, delivering clear directives on delicate topics including personal hygiene. Indigo clarified by stating, "The language, whatever the topic is, our language is just raw. It's what it is. We just speak . . . that's just us as Black mothers, I don't have time. I'm not sugarcoating it. When it comes down to his safety, you got to be raw about it." According to Indigo, Black mothers' communication is direct because of their sons' safety, which is always a matter of urgency. She further explained that Black mothers cannot sugarcoat messages to sons, as the world does not cut Black men slack (Davis, 2018; Houston, 2000; King & Mitchell, 1995; Smitherman, 1986). Indigo held Poobie accountable for his personal hygiene and did not refrain from directly addressing the sensitive topic of body odor with him. She shared:

> I'm raising a Black boy. [Right now] hygiene is his problem. There's manly odors emanating from him. There's also a difference in how we raise our children with disabilities because there's a real-life reality that we don't have the luxury of not exposing them to how we talk. Other moms of other cultures would probably be appalled at the way I talk to him sometimes, but we don't have time to babysit the reality of being a young Black man growing up in this world. He is going to have a function in this world. That odor could cause an interaction with an authority that could be a problem for him. I got to fix that. He got to understand. So, "go handle that" became the mantra for handling personal hygiene. Our code is "go handle that." He knows, you're not going to impose your body on me. Not going to happen.

While maternal concerns regarding adolescent hygiene are not new, BAMs recognized how poor hygiene can translate into politicized matters, as Black males are susceptible and vulnerable to stereotypes regarding self-care. Such stereotypes are also extended to Black mothers and held as value judgments of their ability to properly parent (Harry et al., 2005). Thus, in her efforts to "fix" Poobie's struggles with personal hygiene, Indigo is attempting to protect him from the dangers of society and help him understand that personal hygiene is a form of self-efficacy and independence. Furthermore, it is important to note that Black autism mothers did not conceptualize autism as a "pass" for low expectations but, instead, adapted high standards for their sons. Said otherwise, autism did not provide an out from mothers' expectations of sons because they realized that at the intersection of race, class, gender, and autism, Black men are still bound by low societal expectations.

"I Don't Want Him to Be the Inheritance"

There exists a paucity of research on adults with autism, specifically, detailed examinations of long-term outcomes (Dudley et al., 2019). Given the research on delayed autism diagnosis, higher rates of misdiagnosis, and struggles to obtain autism services, it stands to reason that more nuanced research of autism across the life span of Black adults is needed, along with the experiences of Black caregivers. Existing research does, however, point to concerning life outcomes (Roux et al., 2015). Black youth with autism, who already teeter on the edge of disconnected services, are even more at risk of losing services as they transition into adulthood. The social, physical, and mental health needs of adults with autism intensify with age, leaving families grappling with the loss of social and adaptive skills gained during K–12 schooling (Clarke et al., 2021).

With regard to living arrangements, national data indicates that young adults with autism primarily reside with families: 87% lived at home and 14% in supervised residential settings. Only 19% of young adults with autism lived independently—the majority of those individuals are White (Roux et al., 2015). Black adults with autism are most likely to reside with family members and have limited access to day programming, sheltered employment, and full-employment opportunities (Marsack & Perry, 2018; Roux et al., 2015; Taylor & Seltzer, 2011). Families providing long-term care contend with high stress levels, depression, social isolation, and physical challenges related to care (Roux et al., 2021).

Black mothers in this study provided narratives that underscore the challenges of adult transitions as mothers contemplated future care, employment, and educational opportunities for their sons. Concerns about future care were also punctuated by consideration of mothers' own health, retirement, and life transitions. Participating mothers faced looming questions about what will become of their sons, a question that weighed especially heavily upon those with teen and adult sons; BAMs accepted that they were responsible for their sons' caregiving into adulthood (Gourdine et al., 2011). Participant Candi framed it best: "I don't want him to be the inheritance; I don't want him to be the burden." They were, however, cognizant of their own mortality and that of husbands/partners and were troubled by the prospect of other family members as caregivers or residential care for their sons.

The possibility of neurotypical children caring for siblings with autism was not necessarily a decision mothers favored, but some were left with little choice and few alternatives for long-term care. Donelle took this into consideration when she thought of Bear's future care, as she realized that he would ultimately become his younger brother's responsibility. The possibility of her younger son as primary caregiver tore at her and led her to question, "How do you make one child responsible for another child? What are we gonna do about Bear?" Specifically, Donelle feared that Bear would end up living in his brother's basement on a pull-out couch, literally and figuratively living in isolation. She did not want caregiving responsibilities stifling the dreams of Bear's younger brother. Her fears were compounded by the fact that she and her husband are now retired and live at a distance from extended family; thus, Bear's younger brother is the only family member positioned to take over caregiving from his parents. Bear's younger brother is also the only other family member with intimate knowledge of his health, moods, skills, and needs—information pertinent to caregiving.

Black autism mothers' concerns were further punctuated by their own health issues, family situations, or retirement status; BAMs walked a fine line between placing caregiving above their own needs (Jones et al., 2019). Thelma, for example, was diagnosed with Stage 3 breast cancer shortly after relocating to Texas. As her cancer battle raged, she gave great thought to her younger sons' care should something happen to her. She realized that family members would not be open to caring for two boys with autism, Elijah, 14, and Solomon, 7, especially given Solomon's behavioral issues. The boys' father could care for them, but she also made sure that her oldest son, Daniel, was positioned to assume caregiving responsibilities. Daniel is in the military and travels the world but accepts that he will need to make adjustments to care for his younger brothers.

Thelma and Daniel speak frequently about plans for the boys, and Daniel even communicated the possibility of taking on caregiving responsibilities to his military superiors.

Caregivers are challenged to balance their desires to transition into different life stages with the needs of their children. As Lisa's children grew older and she pondered what her life would entail, she longed to travel and pursue other personal interests. Future considerations, however, were always tempered by concerns about John's ongoing needs. She further elaborated:

> I still worry about what we're going to be doing later, because you sort of want to transition into a different department of your life. Now as I'm moving onto the next stage, where my little one is getting more and more self-sufficient and doesn't need Mom quite as much, and I'm sort of looking for some opportunities to do some different things, and to travel, and to try some new stuff, and what does that look like as far as figuring out how to situate John in a way that makes me feel comfortable.

She realized that balancing the two facets of her life was difficult because John still needed her assistance with daily activities and could not live independently.

Sons' Independence at the Intersection of Race, Class, Gender, and Autism

Most study participants wanted their sons to achieve some semblance of independence based on their individual skill sets. Just as no two individuals on the autism spectrum are alike, BAMs perceptions of independence depended on their sons' communication, social, and behavioral skill sets. For example, Indigo believed Poobie could ultimately live on his own, but in close proximity to the family; however, she still struggled with how Poobie's independence could be actualized. As Poobie prepared to graduate high school, Indigo worried about postsecondary independence, saying, "We are trying to figure out what [independence] means for him." Her vision of independence involves the possibility of their moving into a ranch-style home, post-retirement, with a separate in-law unit, an arrangement that will require the family to finance remodeling or moving to a new home. Indigo, however, believed this option would allow Poobie to live independently but within reach of his parents to provide some assistance. Indigo's example also demonstrates how the actualization of independence for adults with autism is often impacted by a family's financial standing, social capital, and ability to create sheltered opportunities for sons (Taylor & Seltzer, 2011). For example, Indigo plans on leveraging her social networks and approach a local college president about an on-campus opportunity for Poobie. "I know the president up at the community college and she's an amazing community activist and engaged. My plan is to get Poobie connected with them." The community college has programs targeting high-functioning students with autism, providing direct academic and social supports. Families with resources have latitudes regarding schooling and work opportunities that help foster independence for their children on the spectrum because they can more readily access resources (Roux et al., 2015).

Donelle was connected with community-based services that provided job training and coaching for Bear. While he held down a job, Donelle remained concerned about what independence could actually entail for Bear, who still deals with anger issues, which necessitates a job coach to regularly check his progress. He possesses some understanding of money and has some conversational skills, but Donelle realized that Bear cannot navigate society without his parents. "He's never had to navigate. He's been sheltered and this isn't an easy world to navigate." She added, "Bear will not be able to navigate getting his utilities, establish a relationship with a landlord, maintaining a household. No." Donelle was proud of his ability to remain employed but realized the limitations of Bear's independence.

The topic of group home residency proved challenging for study participants, as the vast majority would not consider those placements for their sons. Their resistance bears out in the research literature as Black adults with autism are less likely to reside in group home settings (Roux et al., 2021). BAMs cited several reasons for caution regarding group home placements, including fears of abuse and mistreatment. The possibility of abuse was disconcerting for several participants, including Lisa, who worried about John's ability to report any group home irregularities. She acknowledged that caring for John is proving to be taxing upon the family, especially with her current struggle of locating after-school care. Long term, she says, "he will always need a caretaker," specifically due to John's behaviors, safety issues, and assistance with toileting. She elaborated by adding: "If I were to send him to like a group home situation, could somebody try to molest him or take advantage of him, because he doesn't have, he's not as verbal and he doesn't have a voice? I'm worried about these things constantly. What could happen to him putting him in a group home or something like that might be a solution, but I think I would just be so fearful, only because he just can't advocate for himself." Despite needing respite, Lisa was firm in her concern for John's safety in a group home environment and believed his needs could best be met on an in-home basis with care responsibilities falling upon the nuclear family. Her concerns are further supported by the research literature, which indicates that parents' willingness to place children in residential settings is predicated upon their children's ability to converse (Roux et al., 2015).

Similar to Lisa, Beverly was hesitant to allow anyone other than herself to care for her 16-year-old son, Marvelous. Her fears largely originated from her professional role as an offender rehabilitation counselor coordinator, where she worked with pedophiles returning from prison to society. Beverly's experiences led her to request female teachers and classroom aides for her son, particularly given Marvelous's toileting needs. She shared how such concerns extended to school transportation because she refused to place Marvelous on the bus when his female matron was absent. On those days, she drove him to school. Beverly's fears also stem from a day when Marvelous was lost twice by after-school caregivers, when he was left at the facility and left in public during a field trip. "He's a big kid. How can you lose a big kid over 6 feet?" The incidents resulted in an investigation and policy changes at the agency.

Mothers also struggled with what a placement would mean for their mothering roles, specifically, harkening back to negative perceptions of Black mothers (Wilson Cooper, 2007). Beverly did not easily trust others with her son, even his father, who made overtures to take full custody. She refused to entertain giving up custody, citing her close relationship and detail-oriented care of Marvelous. She expressed these sentiments when addressing the possibilities of his long-term care: "Nobody's going to care for him like I could. So, I need to be there. I'm the kind of person that needs to have hands on and look at that [pointing toward Marvelous]; that's mine. I did that with all my kids. I raised all my kids. I need to be there."

When discussing the possibility of a future group home placement, Beverly was adamant that a placement was not an option for Marvelous. She elaborated:

> I couldn't picture my life without him. I'm like what would I do? Oh my god, that's my sidekick. His father and me is separated; he wants me to give [Marvelous] to him so he can raise him. He must be crazy. I don't be having babies to drop them off. I couldn't do that. I couldn't give up none of my kids. I'm his mother, and I need to be here. He makes my value. I'm rushing home from work to go get my son. Like what would I do? What would I do if he wasn't there? I'd probably get another job. No. He needs me. He looks forward to me. We have a routine. I need him. He's my right hand. That's my right hand. I love him.

Giving the responsibility of Marvelous's care to someone else was tantamount to abandonment, according to Beverly, because she built her life around him and refused to think of life without him in close proximity. Marvelous's care was a point of deep pride and in some ways served as an affront to stereotypes of Black mothers as uncaring and unreasonably difficult (Wilson Cooper, 2009).

While each mother's circumstances differed, the hesitancy to consider residential placements or assisted living arrangements for their sons was a common theme across participants as they considered future care options. The decision to place sons in residential or assisted living is an individual choice and not one that is easily made. Placements may be contingent upon a variety of factors, including individualized medical and safety concerns, social needs, the availability of placements, and familial circumstances (Dudley et al., 2019). The decision for Black autism mothers, however, is further complicated by the sociohistorical and political contexts of Black motherhood. Participants spoke at length about how Black mothers are pathologized, criminalized, and maligned across education, health, and social systems (Collins, 1994; Richie, 1999). Thus, Black mothers' resistance to group home placements may actually be an enactment of motherwork, with BAMs exercising protective love to counter hegemonic forces of racial trauma and discrimination (Chapman & Bhopal, 2013; Collins, 1994; Wilson Cooper, 2007). Residential care, whether full-time or assisted, may be viewed as surrendering a child to the very systems that work against Black families' interests and well-being. The lingering impact of racial trauma may then have some bearing on a family's decision to seek long-term care outside the home, as maintaining intact family care circles is important to people who historically were separated and subjected to violence and abuse (Jones et al., 2019).

Black autism mothers also represented a dichotomy of care, with Black mothers resisting much-needed caregiving assistance at a personal cost to their health, well-being, and long-term aspirations (Bryant-Davis & Ocampo, 2005; Corbin et al., 2018). The dichotomy operationalizes the superwoman trope, a long-standing metaphorical representation of Black women's strength and sacrifice (Avent Harris, 2019; Woods-Giscombe, 2010; Woods-Giscombe et al., 2019). Black women sacrifice personal well-being, taking on additional stress, for collective cultural interests. For example, Black caregivers may not seek help, believing that help-seeking exposes "family business" making them vulnerable to outside scrutiny (Jones et al., 2019). Black caregivers, as noted in the research literature, instead rely on family and faith as coping mechanisms when providing long-term caregiving for adults with disabilities (Kolomer et al., 2002; Tarakeshwar & Pargament, 2001).

Chapter Summary

Participating mothers spoke of fears regarding long-term care for their sons, with some reservations regarding placement with family members, as they did not want their sons to burden anyone. Mothers of younger sons had not yet started to think about long-term care and instead focused more broadly upon developing "good Black men" who challenged societal preconceptions about Black men. BAMs were cognizant of how negative social perceptions of Black men were further compounded by their sons' autism diagnosis. In response, participating mothers purposefully spoke positivity into their sons' lives and emphasized their strengths. Preparation for adulthood evolved around maintaining culturally grounded high behavioral expectations including household duties, personal hygiene, self-care, and socialization.

The future weighed heavily on mothers of teen and adult sons as they worried about caregiving in light of their own life circumstances, including retirement, illness, and even death. Consistent with the research on Black caregivers of adults with autism, participating mothers accepted long-term caregiving responsibilities. BAMs were hesitant to place sons in residential care due to fears of mistreatment and abuse that sons may not be able to fully communicate. In turn, they prepared other siblings, sometimes reluctantly, to take on caregiving responsibilities in the event of their demise. Black mothers' positioning in sociohistorical and political contexts may also influence BAMs perspectives on residential care with mothers opting to maintain care within family structures.

Conclusion

Fast-forward a few years and we fell into a regular Sunday routine of weekly visits to Caleb's group home. Church at 10:00, a coffee run, followed by the hour-long drive to his rural home. On the way, Husband and I engage in our Caleb preparation routine. Satellite radio stays on our favorite gospel channel, although occasionally we forget and are reminded by Caleb repeating inappropriate song lyrics. (Such incidents remind me of the time in second grade when he recited the lyrics of a popular Ludacris song to a teacher who invaded his space, "Get back, get back, you don't know me like that.")

We discuss in advance the words of wisdom we intend to share with him during our visit. If we received any troubling news from school regarding behaviors, the words of wisdom relate specifically to those behaviors and strategies to avoid repeating those behaviors. We use our visits to teach him how to advocate for himself, pouring confidence into him with recognition for positive choices. Our words follow a consistent theme of self-respect, good hygiene, good decision-making, and self-pride. The lessons in self-respect are typically conveyed through my husband's stories of interactions with his students in his school administrator role. Such stories are an effective communication tool with Caleb, 17, as he can make judgments about the behaviors of others easier than he can apply the same rules to his own behaviors. A story about a food fight, leaving school without authorization, or other poor decisions made by adolescent boys typically yield a reply of "Gee, that was pretty stupid" from Caleb.

Lessons in self-pride include references to Black history or current events with a direct impact on Black America. He looks forward to these conversations and prepares in advance by watching CNN. We want him to have knowledge of self, along with the ability to share his knowledge with his peers. Our weekly visits also provide a much-needed release of his political views. As the lone Black male in his classes, I worry about how others relate to him, most certainly, his political views. He lives in rural America where it is not unusual to see Confederate flags flying on the back of pickup trucks or posted in the front window of a dilapidated house occupied by a classmate. He is sensitive to how his views are received by peers. Thus, he bounces ideas off us, ideas he has learned are not welcome in his school environment. I often wonder how he developed the sense of what's safe and unsafe to say, while yet again, worrying about the fact that he has to self-sensor in an environment where his views are widely divergent.

On one Sunday visit, our 4-year-old granddaughter accompanied us to see her uncle. She is still too young to understand his living arrangements but, nonetheless, is nonplussed by his presence. Caleb is always delighted to see Laylah, whom he believes is a connection to her father, my stepson, who now resides in Texas. He takes his role of uncle seriously and believes he has a responsibility to teach her life lessons. I marvel at the depths of his love for her as demonstrated through his words and actions. He always shares stories of her birth, which he missed because he was away at camp. He tells her the story of how he dug up a rubber duck buried in the yard, carefully cleaned it, and then gifted it to her. He is truly at his best around her.

We headed to our standard restaurant where the server knows us by name and our orders by heart. In between rounds of soda, Husband blessed the food. Laylah then asked us, with the curiosity of a 4-year-old, "Who is Jesus?" Before we could answer, Caleb immediately took the lead and explained to her in age-appropriate language, "Well Laylah, Jesus is a great guy who loves all of us. He wants us to be good people, help our neighbors, and love each other. He died to make us better people. He's who we pray to." Laylah listened intently and then asked, "What's pray?" Using his hands to demonstrate, he replied, "Well, it's when you have something in your heart that you only want Jesus to know. So, you write Jesus a letter. A prayer is a letter from your heart to Jesus."

Husband and I sat with our mouths open, amazed by the depths of his faith and his ability to convey his beliefs to his 4-year-old niece. Okay, you preach Caleb. Laylah responded, "Okay," then popped a French fry into her mouth. We spent the rest of our meal asking Caleb to elaborate on his ideas. Moreover, we sat with pride at this loving faith-filled young man. I listen and I am reminded of how parents play such a vital role in shaping the lives of their children by preparing them for the world. My mother used to describe such efforts as "I'm doing the best I can with what I got" to prepare me for life. Caleb respects elders, exercises faith, and loves family. These qualities will help him be successful in the future. I am Caleb's mom, and I am enough.

∽

This final chapter discusses key points from across the text, seeking to make further sense of Black autism mothers' experiences mothering at the intersection of race, class, gender, and autism. As such, the format of this chapter offers a more interactive conversational flow, with sections summarizing specific arguments and targeted points for specific groups. As noted at the beginning of the book, the intent is not to provide "magic bullet" checklists for those interested in working with Black autism families. In my professional work with teachers and leaders, I rebuke the practice of boiling down important concepts into inconsequential to-do lists that can then be interpreted as completed tasks. Doing so precludes authentic "dungeon-shaking" work, that is, the creation of engaging learning experiences, which author James Baldwin described as creating a profound shift in one's reality, thought processes, and actions. Thus, the danger of checklists is the creation of simplistic responses to complex social problems at the intersection of race, class, gender, and autism that launch immediately to superficial action, versus a shift in consciousness needed for deep, abiding change.

Follow-up questions are used as a means of dungeon shaking or consciousness shifting. Holding up the mirror to oneself can be a healthy means of examining one's beliefs, particularly coupled with narratives that produce seismic change: "Any upheaval in the universe is terrifying because it so profoundly attacks one's sense of one's own reality" (Baldwin, 1993, p. 9). The narratives featured in this book may have elicited a similar response from readers, leaving some wanting to take direct action steps. Or other readers may still be questioning why a book on Black autism mothers is necessary when all mothers of autistic children manage challenging behaviors, attend IEP meetings, as well as wrangle with service providers and myriads of medical appointments.

The difference lies in understanding the motherwork of Black autism mothers, who are fighting for their sons' survival in systems steeped in anti-Black racism (Collins, 1994, 2016). At the intersection of race, class, gender, and autism, Black autism mothers, despite class standing and educational levels, must still battle for services in systems that center whiteness (Straiton & Sridhar, 2022; Stahmer et al., 2019). Black autism mothers are not just mothers but are perceived as Black women in autism spaces by autism service providers, educators, and other autism mothers. Said otherwise, BAMs are accompanied into these spaces by generations of misconceptions of Black mothers and negative stereotypes held of Black women, placing them at a deficit while navigating autism spaces. Their presence is not race, class, or gender neutral. BAMs across the text describe strategies used to counter such notions and low expectations held of them. In addition to societal expectations for Black mothers, Black sons, despite the presence of autism, are still subjected to low educational outcomes and criminal expectations. Black autism mothers' identities, and perceptions of their identities and that of their Black autistic sons, impact daily facets of life. My hope is that readers have listened intently to their narratives for a better understanding of how Black mothers and sons' identities are inseparable at the intersection of race, class, gender, and autism (Annamma et al., 2013).

Revisiting Conceptualizations of Autism Mothers

I began the book with a discussion of pervasive conceptualizations of autism mothering as a space occupied by White middle- to upper middle-class women. Autism mothering is a form of warrior mothering, with White mothers combatting autism from the root causes, the treatment, and the goal of autism eradication (Chivers Yochim & Silva, 2013; Douglas, 2013). By centering White women as the standard of autism motherhood, the erroneous presumption that race does not matter in autism is reinforced. Black women's motherwork is connected to the survival of Black people, providing a means to understand how and why participating Black autism mothers utilized their personal experiences, social capital, and professional expertise in advocacy (Collins, 1994). It is from this understanding of Black motherhood that participating Black mothers in this study described autism advocacy, not as a singular transactional endeavor with individualistic end goals. BAMs are not without agency and relied heavily upon their Christian faith for empowerment. According to participants, advocacy was not a choice, per se, but a spiritual mission in which they enacted the faith that empowered them. BAMs felt called to share knowledge, leverage professional connections, and even create nonprofits to share with other Black families.

In some ways, participating BAMs are arguing for expanded autism cultural spaces with greater recognition that autism impacts Black families as well (Douglas, 2013). The term autism spaces, in the case of mothers in this study, refers to autism nonprofit organizations that provide services for families and individuals, autism health care providers, and schools, including the IEP process. BAMs also referred to public images and perceptions of autism. Finally, BAMs referred to Black families, Black churches, and society writ large as spaces where greater autism visibility is needed for Black autism families. The term expanded autism spaces, however, builds upon expanding ideas of who is *autistic*, who represents the face(s) of autism, and recognition that families' autism narratives are socially situated. This notion implies that the autism journey, diagnosis, treatments, schooling, services, adult transitions, and other key stages are socially situated in racial, gendered, and classed contexts. These contexts result in varied responses to autism from families, as demonstrated by the Black autism mothers in this study. For example, a few BAMs in this study reported feeling excluded from autism organizations and the realization that popular autism treatments were out of reach due to financial limitations.

Expanding autism cultural spaces also calls for an examination of how hegemonic forces benefit White autism families while marginalizing families of color, those geographically isolated from autism resources, and low-income families. A realization of how White families hold power within autism communities and the ways in which others are excluded requires a nuanced intersectional examination, doing what DiAngelo (2018) suggests is a hard examination of White fragility and privilege. BAMs were cognizant of White autism mothers, but most participants had limited or no interactions with White peers. Nor did they go out of their way to meet White mothers or interact with them, with the exception of the mothers involved in nonprofit work. In those instances, interactions with White autism mothers and members of the White autism community were leveraged to learn about autism resources and share that information with other Black families. It is important to note, however, that mothers in this study described few instances of White autism mothers making overtures to them. Thus, their experiences speak to racial and gendered divisions within the autism community, thereby challenging the notion of an autism "community." As highlighted in chapter 5, however, BAMs maintained hope and espoused beliefs regarding culturally responsive practices—cultural competence, sociocultural awareness, and high expectations—for autism services providers. Organizations can make inroads into communities of color and bilingual communities by locating key figures and institutions within those communities. The void of Black autism mothers at decision-making tables was highlighted by participants who brought a wealth of personal and professional experiences to leadership tables, if provided opportunities to serve. A close analytical read of BAMs' narratives also provides starting points for those seeking to provide culturally responsive services incorporating cultural competence, sociopolitical consciousness, and high expectations (Gay, 2010; Ladson-Billings, 1995; Pearson & Meadan, 2021). Organizations must make deliberate efforts to invite Black and brown mothers into their settings—as board members, partaking in services, sponsoring scholarships for their children to participate in autism events, and bringing services to communities of color.

BAMs also expressed a willingness to participate in autism research while noting the lack of Black families in autism research (Cascio et al., 2021; Jones & Mandell, 2020; Shaia et al., 2020; Yee, 2016). Most of all, providers should not presume to know their needs or make assumptions that their needs mirror those of White parents or families in affluent communities (Stahmer et al., 2019). As demonstrated across this book, Black mothers situated at the matrix of autism, gender, race, and class have distinct experiences with autism service providers that impact diagnosis, treatment, and long-term care. I also encourage researchers to further examine the experiences of Black families and individuals with autism across the life span. This work can further be enhanced by exploring the experiences of Black autism fathers (Hannon & Hannon, 2017; Hannon et al., 2018) or examining the lives of Black women and girls on the spectrum (Lovelace et al., 2021).

Intersectional Considerations for Specific Groups

In the following section, discussion and questions for consideration are presented by specific groups that have been addressed across the book. Groups include Black families, churches and houses of worship, educators, autism providers (including human service and medical professionals), and Black autism mothers (BAMs). Again, the questions are intended to provoke thought and conversation on an individual basis, in pairs, and within organizations.

BLACK AUTISM MOTHERS

My hope is that this book will spark discussions and move BAMs to action across the nation. As demonstrated by the BAMs in this book, the autism diagnosis moved them to action in various forms, including special needs ministries, online chat groups, sharing information with other Black autism mothers, and the establishment of nonprofits. These are examples of advocacy that made sense to the participants or, as they highlighted, advocacy that originated from a spiritual call. The call may look different for readers across various communities because the needs may vary.

In your community, the needs of Black autism mothers may center on connecting BAMs to services by means of service fairs located within Black communities or at Black churches. BAMs can raise autism awareness in Black communities by hosting autism information Sundays with guest speakers from local autism organizations or the medical community. This serves the dual purpose of providing these constituents entry into Black community spaces, facilitating connections. BAMs might start out small, hosting small gatherings in homes, spaces where their children can interact, reminiscent of study participant Marley's description of an "autism house."

Self-care is a critical dimension to the lives of caregivers, for without attention to self, the possibility of losing oneself becomes real. Black autism mothers across this study provided examples of self-care, from reading, worship/Bible study, painting nails, to enjoying hot baths. Self-care was a means of exercising self-compassion needed to sustain caregiving responsibilities and to maintain life balance. The point is that participating mothers realized that they must care for themselves in order to care for others. One mother, for example, took yearly vacations with her other children not only to relax but also to provide a break for the children, as they were a critical part of the caregiving circle. Readers are encouraged to examine their self-care regimen to remain prepared to undertake caregiving, employment, family, and other community-related responsibilities. The participants were able to "make lemonade" and create full lives for themselves and their sons.

I encourage BAMs to take bold steps and push into places where Black autism mothers have seemingly been over-excluded, including autism research (Cascio et al., 2021; Maye et al., 2022; Steinbrenner et al., 2022). There are numerous opportunities to participate in autism studies at research centers across the country, but researchers must intentionally include Black families. Researchers must understand that intersections of race, class, gender, and other identities impact how families access autism services and long-term autism outcomes. Quantitative studies may call for the completion of instruments assessing autism-related behaviors, treatments, or genome research, but I challenge researchers to think beyond paradigmatic comfort zones to pose research questions that require a variety of methodological approaches. The presence of BAMs is most certainly needed in qualitative studies, as we must begin to describe autism from our standpoint, noting the particularities of our experiences. I do, however, caution BAMs to select studies that align with your personal values. (For example, some mothers may decline participation in studies focused on identifying autism causes with the purpose of eradicating autism.) To date, I have participated in two autism studies, one of which I seemingly forced my way into by reminding the researchers that Black families could enhance the data. The researchers conceded and ultimately used some of my data in a publication. Thus, if BAMs do not participate, our autism narratives will continue to be framed by White mothers' experiences with services and treatments built upon research in which we are invisibilized.

In conducting this research, I wanted BAMs to become aware that they are not alone. Meeting the participants, even those who could not participate in the study, provided me with the opportunity to meet other BAMs that I would have never interacted with in other capacities. Moreover, the study emphasizes that BAMs have collective narratives marked by a process of acceptance, challenges, advocacy, fears, mission work, moments of levity, and concerns about the impact of race, class, gender, and autism on their sons. In reading this book, my hope is that other Black autism mothers can identify with the collective experiences presented, as I have sought to center the particularities of our standpoints within the larger autism conversation. As such, I pose the following questions for BAMs:

- How are you exercising self-care?
- Are you pleased with your son's current level of autism supports? If not, what are the barriers to improved care levels? Do you have a service care coordinator?

- In what ways can you share your experiences with other Black autism mothers?

- In what ways can you share your experiences with the broader autism community if you have not attempted to do so already?

- Mothers in this study were asked to provide recommendations and insights to autism providers, including medical, therapeutic, human services, and educational. If provided the opportunity to share with your son's providers, what recommendations would you make?

- BAMs shared fears and concerns surrounding raising Black sons with autism. What fears and concerns do you have regarding raising your son at the intersection of race, class, gender, and autism?

- Based on your reading of the book, what is your action plan?

Black Families

Participating BAMs offered varying pictures of family supports and caregiving contributions. Black autism mothers conceptualize the autism journey as pictures of action. Black families figured prominently in these pictures, with BAMs acquiring and sharing autism knowledge with husbands/partners and other family members. The family constellation, along with mothers' faith, was essential to mothers' mental well-being across the autism journey. While the literature on kinship and Black families stresses how they provide a collective-centered safety net, mothers in this study confronted family members with contrasting behaviors (Stack & Burton, 2016). They described feeling lonely, judged, and misunderstood due to their sons' autism, as their families did not understand autism. The lack of understanding translated into hostility, resentment, and familial disconnection from mothers and their sons. BAMs longed for family interactions with their sons, as one participant described how her family never babysat or invited her son to family birthday parties. Such interactions proved hurtful to participants.

The takeaway message for Black families is that collective support matters in the lives of BAMs. For example, I shared in the introduction that a close family member pointed out signs of autism in my son. With her guidance, I was able to take the first steps toward seeking a diagnosis and early intervention services. This incident demonstrates that family ties of trust can make a difference in when Black children are diagnosed (Stahmer et al., 2019). If autism expertise exists in families, those members must speak up and share their insights in helpful versus scornful ways. Support of young mothers in this situation is particularly crucial, as they may rely upon familial insight and opinions for guidance in child rearing.

The autism journey as articulated by BAMs also included an autism learning curve. In my own experience, the autism journey included educating family members about autism, responding to their questions regarding behaviors in real time. And, similar to the mothers in this study, I learned to push pride and guilt aside, refocus on my son, teach others, and ask for help. Posing questions to BAMs and even their sons, if reasonable, is a powerful means of opening up minds and hearts to challenging discussions regarding autism. Families can also take the initiative to learn more about autism by recognizing what they do not know. There is a growing presence of Black parents and families sharing their stories across social media platforms (Morgan & Stahmer, 2020). The autism learning curve presents an opportunity for family members to learn in sync with BAMs, demonstrating support and a genuine interest in autism. Gains in autism knowledge can also help further autism discussions within families, as members can therefore build a shared discourse incorporating established autism terms and terms translated into the family's idioms.

BAMs transitioned through feelings of guilt and encouragement to a point where most could figuratively "make lemonade" out of lemons. The proximity of family members is important, as they have the ability to reassure mothers struggling to locate services, dealing with autism-related behaviors, or managing self-doubt. My mother's words, "You are doing the best you can with what you have," resounded in my ears frequently as I blamed myself for Caleb's struggles in school and community settings. Her words were instrumental in lifting me from guilt to encouragement and ultimately helped me become more determined to establish a new "normal" along the way. Families must realize that an encouraging word can be a powerful lifter during challenging times. An offer of lunch, an hour of babysitting, an offer to shop for a BAM, or a listening ear are ways to demonstrate support for BAMs in your family. Or, as one participant highlighted, developing a means of maintaining schedules and rewards systems for autistic family members during visits greatly assists BAMs in transitioning their children across settings.

Black families must also understand that autism caregiving is a lifelong endeavor as youth transition into adulthood. The transition into adulthood for individuals with autism is also marked by a disconnect from autism services including physical health, mental health, and social programming (Hendricks & Wehman, 2009). Employment and independent living prospects for adults with autism depend greatly on communication abilities and access to community-based services (Roux et al., 2015, 2021). Given the challenges of adult transitions, the need for familial support intensifies as Black autism parents must make future plans and caregiving arrangements. For a variety of reasons, Black autism mothers in this study did not consider group home placements or assisted living a viable option for their sons' long-term care, setting in motion back-up plans for husbands/partners and neurotypical children to assume caregiving responsibilities in the event of their demise or illness.

Family members of BAMs are encouraged to reflect upon the following questions:

- How did you first learn about autism?
- In what ways have you been supportive of BAMs within your family? In what ways can you improve upon demonstrating support for them?
- In what ways have you been supportive of family members with autism? In what ways can you improve upon demonstrating support for autistic family members?
- How have you increased your knowledge of autism?
- Hold a conversation with a BAM in your family about managing autism-related behaviors, schooling issues, advocacy, and self-care. What insights were gained? How can insights from an autism mother change the way in which you interact with your family members?

Churches and Houses of Worship

Participants in this study identified as Christians and most maintained congregational memberships. Several participants described feeling ostracized and unwelcome as they navigated congregational dynamics in churches that did not understand autism. Black church leaders must recognize how autism impacts Black families and develop ways of welcoming and involving Black autism families into congregations. Church school instructors must also find ways to include autistic children in the hallmarks of Black church youth programming, including weekly church school classes and annual church plays. The autism knowledge of Black autism mothers like Candi and Ginger, who also led special needs Christian education classes, should be tapped to help churches create autism-friendly approaches to ministry. Black churches could also provide a cultural space for Black autism families by hosting autism awareness events, trainings, and creating social media content highlighting church-based autism strategies.

Mothers did not refrain from bringing their sons to worship and found ways to be included as Sunday school teachers in classes for special needs children. In doing so, they pushed back on social expectations of exclusion, silence of autistic children, and the larger message of marginalization. Instead, they navigated church power structures and filled a need that the churches did not necessarily recognize as a need until the mothers came forward to work with special needs children. With the increasing numbers of Black children with autism, Black churches, which have long been considered a bulwark in Black communities and sites of political action, must step forward to intentionally create welcoming environments for autism families. Churches should offer training for church officers and those in the help ministries, especially ushers and church greeters. These are typically the first faces that visitors and members see upon entering a church building and thus can send a message of welcome to autism families.

Sometimes, churches need to assess whether or not they are inclusive or restrictive to members and visitors with special needs. As demonstrated by study participants, Black mothers want to attend church and bring their autistic children with them. The church environment can prove daunting for some children on the spectrum with sensory issues. For example, music is an important form of praise in Black churches. But for autistic children, the clashing of cymbals, tambourines, the organ, and other praise-yielding instruments may lead to sensory overload. Noise-canceling headphones available to members or visiting families would allow them to stay in church longer. Sound/lighting ministries should also be cognizant that flashing lights can trigger behavioral responses in children with autism.

Churches might well consider revisiting rigid restrictions on children reading and using technology during church. One mother in this study, for example, transitioned her son into church services by using headphones, a tablet, or her laptop, allowing her son to watch Christian-themed movies and cartoons. If available, churches may think about creating autism spaces, where children or adults with autism can go to decompress if they become too overstimulated during a service. The larger point is that autism mothers, as expressed in this study, want judgment-free spaces where they can worship, participate, and be accepted.

Churches may consider identifying members with autism expertise to welcome autism families into the church, shepherd them through the various ministries, and intercede on their behalf with members who lack an understanding of autism. Families need members who can support them while they participate in various ministries such as ushering or choir. One mother in this study, for example, strategically seats her son up front, on the same pew as two church trustees. These gentlemen are reasonably versed in autism and the young man responds well to them. This allows the mother an opportunity to participate in the choir, a ministry that she finds fulfilling. She took the time to converse with the two trustees and other members who regularly sit near her son, explaining his behaviors and appropriate responses to him.

Mothers may also consider creating or adapting a social story on church for their autistic children. I searched online for church-related social stories and located a few related to Catholic Church services and activities. The stories targeted children in younger age ranges. These stories could serve as a basis for adaptation to social expectations and practices across faiths. For example, social stories can be used to introduce children to expectations for church behaviors, such as sitting and standing; introduce them to individuals with key roles; and prepare them for the general worship atmosphere. Mothers may also want to consider meeting with the pastor in advance to assess their understanding of autism and how receptive the ministerial staff is to learn more about autism. In doing so, they may learn that other church members have children or adults on the spectrum. I encourage churches and worship centers to consider the following questions:

- How can you assess if your church is a welcoming atmosphere for parents and individuals with autism?
- In what ways do your existing church ministries encourage or limit participation of families or individuals with autism?
- Do you have any members with autism within your congregation? If so, how can you learn from these families?

- How can you share their knowledge of autism, or utilize their knowledge to increase autism awareness within your congregation? Is there a specific day of community service, part of a Sunday service, or school recess time during which you can educate families on autism symptoms, diagnosis, and services available in your community?

- If you do not have autism resources, what ministries within the church can commit to seeking out autism resources and introducing said resources to the church body?

- Can you identify willing volunteers to function as members of an autism welcome team?

- How can you designate church resources for the needs of autistic church members and their families?

Autism Providers and Educators

During the first portion of the book, I noted the disparities between White and Black children diagnosed with autism. Black children are diagnosed at later ages and misdiagnosed at higher rates than their White peers (Constantino et al., 2020; Mandell & Novak, 2005). While this fact has been discussed in the autism literature, BAMs still have concerns regarding medical care received, particularly that at autism clinics. Several mothers critiqued autism services due to lengthy diagnosis processes and appointments that provided little to no practical information related to autism services (Moh & Magiati, 2012). The asymmetrical power relationship between medical providers and BAMs can also translate into mistrust, especially when factoring a history of mistrust toward the medical community (Carr & Lord, 2012; Delgado Rivera & Rogers-Atkinson, 1997; Leininger, 1991; Leininger & McFarland, 2007; Nickerson et al., 1994; Washington, 2006). Thus, it is important for autism medical professionals to demonstrate some level of cultural competence when working with Black families, and especially when interacting with Black autism mothers. BAMs want to be heard and have their experiences factored into treatment plans. Doing so recognizes Black mothers' autism expertise and demonstrates a consideration of socioeconomics on the decisions Black families make related to care, education, and services. BAMs in this study also mentioned feeling judged and scrutinized. Medical professionals may be able to counteract such negative forces with recognition of BAMs' mothering skills and acumen.

For educators, it is important to note that Black children, upon diagnosis, are more likely to receive autism services in public school settings as opposed to private care settings (Siller, Reyes, et al., 2013). This is not surprising given the ability of White parents to leverage public resources supplemented by private resources (Dixson et al., 2015). This fact further emphasizes the importance of service quality and quantity received in school-based settings. I also reviewed the precarious relationships Black mothers often have with schools. The book described how, historically, relationships between Black mothers and schools have been troubled by mothers' previous schooling experiences and larger societal subjugation of Black women, leaving them invisibilized and unheard. BAMs exercised advocacy, where they were able to speak power over their sons and themselves. As such, they had a better grasp of the autism landscape and a recognition that the journey was continuous.

Advocacy was also evidenced in BAMs confronting service providers (chapter 4) and educators (chapter 5) over missteps. Motherwork informs how Black women approach school advocacy as a political act, as they recognize their actions benefit not only their child but Black children collectively (Collins, 1994, 2016). Black autism mothers engaged in motherwork, a form of Black women's motherhood that challenged stereotypes and pathologizing of Black mothers (Wilson Cooper, 2007). This facet of motherwork empowered Black mothers, leading them to strategize on how to access information, a form of social capital (Wilson Cooper, 2007). Black autism mothers strategized regarding whom to bring to the special education table—the negotiation space for resources that will determine long-term outcomes for their sons.

Motherwork also undergirded Black autism mothers' advocacy for fair treatment and high expectations, as they pushed educators to move beyond stigma to service. While BAMs collectively reported microaggressions and resentment to their advocacy, they also shared examples of how they partnered with schools to ensure positive learning outcomes for their sons. As educated middle-class women, study participants astutely recognized that autism knowledge translated into a form of social capital that they drew upon to access autism services in schools and communities.

As educators, it is important to recognize that Black autism mothers have agency, and the ability to determine the educational course for their children. The mothers in this study demonstrated a keen recognition that education is not simply for today but has lasting implications for the future. BAMs expressed concerns regarding classroom and school placements that can determine life outcomes. Black autism mothers also come to the special education table prepared to present the best well-rounded picture of their sons. One participant, for example, balked at the use of "violent" to describe her son's behavior and refused to sign any paperwork until the term was removed. Mothers want educators to recognize that their sons have futures that BAMs are greatly vested in by virtue of high expectations, political action, and advocacy.

A common sentiment across BAMs was negative perceptions of them that interfered with gaining or continuing much-needed supports for their sons. In the case of several mothers, teachers and support staff were heard making disparaging comments regarding BAMs. One case, in particular, highlighted educators stepping outside their prescribed roles, making undiagnosed determinations for her son. These scenarios and others demonstrate that BAMs want educators to collaborate with them on seeking quality services delivered by caring adults in a safe school environment (Stoner et al., 2005). BAMs, however, also articulated that they wanted educators to understand their roles and to do their jobs. Said otherwise, if a teacher is assigned to teach special education, then they should be a resource to the child and parents. The focus should remain on the child and not on negative perceptions of Black mothers.

Multiple phone calls home with complaints regarding the child's behavior are not helpful, as one participant articulated, as BAMs are looking to educators to be the professionals. In doing so, a caveat should be made that BAMs want educators to stay in their professional roles, as opposed to delivering a diagnosis they are neither trained nor equipped to make. One mother was adamant about this point when a teacher attempted to make a psychological diagnosis of her child. Such actions contribute to the cycle of parental mistrust, leading Black mothers to question educators' intentions—did they intend to harm or benefit the child?

Educators can be of great assistance to families of children with autism by exercising the principles of cultural relevance—sociopolitical consciousness, high standards/academic expectations, and cultural competence. As reviewed in this book, cultural relevance provides a framework for educators to utilize when interacting with Black families, particularly those with children with special needs such as autism. Take the time to read, particularly in the areas of culturally responsive/culturally relevant work (Gay, 2010; Ladson-Billings, 1995); establishing cooperative relationships with families that are linguistically and racially diverse (Harry, 2007; Pearson & Meadan, 2021); and the developing field of DisCrit, which examines the intersection of race and disability (Annamma et al., 2013). Medical providers, autism service providers, and educators may want to consider the following questions:

- What are your perceptions of Black mothers? What are your perceptions of Black mothers based upon?

- Based upon your reading of this text, what issues emerge as important to BAMs? Specifically, educational issues? Health care issues? Autism services, including therapies?

- Based upon your reading of this text, how do you now understand the critical nature of parent–teacher relationships? In what ways have your perceptions of Black mothers shifted or remained the same?

- What is the role of teachers in the CSE process? What is the role of administrators? Support professionals, including occupational therapy (OT), speech, and physical therapy (PT)? Based upon your reading of the text, in what ways would the participating mothers agree or disagree with your role descriptions?

- For medical professionals, how does your professional role factor into the autism journey as described by BAMs across this text?

- Describe your current practices when working with families of children on the autism spectrum. In what ways can this book inform your practices, particularly when interacting with parents of different racial and linguistic backgrounds?

Law Enforcement

Black autism mothers recognized that Black males are adultified, criminalized, and seen as threats by law enforcement and society writ large. In one unfortunate incident, a participating mother's worst fears were actualized when her son was attacked by a White man, who initially went unpunished. Another participant's son was subjected to bullying while his assailants were unpunished by school authorities. The instance also demonstrated the leveraging of law enforcement to silence a participant who sought answers to the bullying.

The precarious relationship between Black men and law enforcement, particularly racial profiling, greatly concerned participating BAMs who worried about how their sons would comply and interact with law enforcement officers. They also worried about resulting actions on the part of law enforcement officers' responses to noncompliance, echolalia, and lack of eye contact. BAMs' fears were reinforced by experiences of husbands and other sons who experienced racial profiling. In turn, Black autism mothers strategized on how best to deliver "the talk" to sons, in an attempt to raise their awareness to racialized violence.

With regard to autism training, law enforcement agencies across the country now engage in training that helps them identify autism-related behaviors (National Autistic Society, 2011). Data is even available on law enforcement officers' knowledge of autism-related behaviors including repetitive motions, lack of eye contact, and noncompliance (Gardner et al., 2019). Officers now are taught to identify these behaviors, particularly when deescalating high anxiety and helping to bring lost children home. While the training is critical to assisting autism families and individuals in crisis, it is delivered with little to no regard for race. For Black men on the autism spectrum, these same behaviors might otherwise be deemed suspicious and filtered through a racialized lens that positions Black men as threats. For example, Debbaudt (2002) developed autism response cards to identify individuals as autistic and provide officers with information on how to interact with the individuals. The idea presumes that officers will take time to review a card versus immediately reacting to a Black male or engaging in racial profiling (Modell & Copp, 2007). Black males have been shot while retrieving wallets from their pockets or due to a phone mistaken as a firearm (Alexander, 2010). Here again is another example of the intersection of race, class, gender, and autism.

My comments do not discount the importance of law enforcement in assisting autism families. In my own experience, I became familiar with officers who returned my son home following wandering incidents. I also saw firsthand how officers in my city worked diligently to locate a Black autistic young man who eloped from school; the young man was later found dead, drowned in a river. These are examples of officers working with autism families with the shared goal of ensuring safety. However, the narratives of BAMs raise additional questions for law enforcement, including:

- Does your agency require autism training? If so, how many hours?

- Does your agency collect data to assess the effectiveness of autism training? If so, what kind of data? What does the data reveal?

- Does your agency currently participate in training that addresses racial profiling and autism awareness simultaneously?

- After reading BAMs' narratives, how can law enforcement better address the intersection of race, class (as determined by neighborhoods), gender, and autism?

- How can your agency directly engage Black autism families as a means of raising autism awareness and cultural responsiveness?

AUTISM ORGANIZATIONS

I have worked with organizations across the years on diversity initiatives, including evaluations, curriculum reviews, curriculum development, and data plans targeting diversity efforts. In doing this work, it is important that organizations begin with open minds regarding their current situations related to diversity and inclusion. Said otherwise, organizations must be willing to name areas of concern, weakness, or strength. The information needed to do so typically comes from frontline staff or from communities that are not currently served by the organization.

While I recognize the varied scales on which autism organizations exist, from small operations to larger entities, much work is needed to shift understandings of autism and who falls under the autism umbrella. For example, participants explained they do not participate in existing autism groups due to geographic distance, the absence of Black families, and pronounced class differences. Taken further, said differences translate into services offered during the day when parents who work full-time cannot attend, transportation issues to and from activities in suburban areas, and participation fees. Black autism mothers, as articulated across this study, are cautious when interacting with autism specialists due to long-standing pathologizing of Black mothers, Black women, and Black families. Autism organizations must develop welcoming pathways for racially, ethnically, linguistically, and socioeconomically diverse families, as they too fall under the large autism umbrella. Furthermore, organizations must sincerely be committed to expanding their reach; otherwise, organizations will continue to only benefit those who created them and members of their social networks.

It is critical for autism organizations to place the mirror in front of themselves to respond to the following questions:

- What is the takeaway message from BAMs that highlights strengths and shortcomings in autism organizations?

- Who is your organization designed to serve? What groups or individuals serve as the focal point of your organization's activities, fundraising, and services?

- What does organizational data reveal regarding primary recipients of your services? Income? Geography? Race? Gender? Caregivers?

- Are you an inclusive organization, meaning, do you offer programming that meets the needs of families across classes? How do you know?

- In what ways does your organization reflect and welcome those you currently serve via optics, that is, your website, frontline staff, midlevel leadership, and board?

- What data sources can you draw upon to inform organizational diversity efforts? Do you have the expertise within your organization to collect such data, particularly within communities and across linguistic communities?

- With regard to organizational leadership, do you have Black board members? Executive and midlevel leadership? Do you have board members and staff from other racial groups representing a cross section of the autism community? If not, why? What organizational barriers have prevented the organization from having a racially and ethnically diverse board or staff?

- In what ways does your organizational mission attend or not attend to issues of race, class, and gender? If not, why not?

In conclusion, this chapter summarized points made across the book, seeking to make additional sense of BAMs' interpretations of raising sons at the intersection of race, class, gender, and autism. The chapter also highlighted specific groups, providing recommendations, points of action, and reflective questions. The afterword provides brief follow-ups on study participants.

Afterword

I reached out to participating Black autism mothers with two purposes in mind. First, I wanted to thank them again for sharing their narratives with me. The testimonies shared included questions BAMs had never been asked along their autism journey, and they too were grateful for the opportunity to write Black mothers into larger autism narratives. My second reason for reaching out to participating BAMs was to provide readers updates on the mothers and sons, as most of the interviews occurred a year prior to writing the text. Black autism mothers continue to engage in pitched battles for culturally responsive autism services. As reported in this afterword, participating Black autism mothers remain steadfast, resilient, and resourceful in addressing their sons' needs.

Although I did not receive updates from Ginger and Indigo, the remaining study participants provided updates on significant life changes since the time of data collection.

Donelle Boston shared that Bear continues employment at a fast-food restaurant. She was especially passionate in detailing shifts in his medical coverage from Medicaid to Medicare, as he received Social Security for 2 years, whereas he received Supplemental Security Income (SSI) in previous years. Bear transitioned to Social Security when Donelle retired 2 years ago and began receiving Social Security benefits. By sharing this information, Donelle wanted parents of younger sons in this study and readers to understand that the autism journey continues through adulthood and the fight for services does not cease. She further emphasized that autism does not go away.

Candi Charles continues to expand her nonprofit. This spring her nonprofit will host a brunch honoring autism caregivers. The nonprofit is marking year 2 of monthly caregiver support meetings. Pappas is in the 11th grade and made merit roll for the first marking period. He is successfully earning credits toward a state-recognized academic diploma. Pappas continues to run; only this year, he was accompanied by his teaching assistant on cross country and community-based 5k runs. Candi reports that he is focusing on 5k races in the community, regionally, and nationally to assist in establishing future social networks when his teammates begin to graduate this year and next year. Pappas has developed an appreciation of media arts, as he serves as the television camera operator in media classes, responsible for the school's daily news program camera work.

Marley Christian reported that Poopy-Doo, now age 7, is doing well in school. He was recently placed in a general education class where he receives push-in special education services. He also participates in a weekly group counseling session at his school. Marley believes that group counseling is helping him better vocalize his feelings and decrease his frustrations. She continues to be a strong presence at the school, where she attempts to help school staff understand his needs as a Black boy with autism. Marley's short-term advocacy goal is to create a support group for mothers of color that also doubles as a play group. She strongly believes such a group is missing from her community and would be a great asset to support parents of color.

Karla Daniels responded with updates on sons Mikey, now age 7, and Andrew, age 13. Mikey is in a first grade 6:1:2 (six students, one teacher, two aides) classroom for students with autism. The smaller classroom setting is a better fit for Mikey, as he is demonstrating fewer behavioral meltdowns. He continues to see a mental health therapist and receives behavioral therapy. Andrew remains in a 6:1:2 placement and is now in seventh grade. Karla reports that he has some new behaviors surrounding his love of art and technology: he insists on bringing the classroom Chromebook home, crying when he cannot use it at school, and taking art supplies from school. Both boys are involved in music lessons and enjoy visits to the local zoo, science center, and children's play museum.

After the unsettling incident at Elijah's school, **Thelma Fox** shared that he is doing well in his new school placement. Thelma recently posted video of him on social media attending his first high school dance. Although he does not socialize with his peers, Thelma accompanied him to the dance and reported that he danced all night. (The video captured a snippet of him dancing to his favorite song, "Wobble," by V.I.C.) Just recently, Thelma fought for a new school placement for Solomon, now age 8. The process was draining, as she shared, but she was able to get

Solomon placed in a school known for success due to its use of small learning communities.

The past year has been challenging for **Kendra Griffin**, as she closed her pharmacy. Never one to sit still, Kendra did not languish in sadness but, instead, created additional opportunities for herself. She now holds several positions as a part-time pharmacist, a pharmacy preceptor, and running her own tax business. Her boys, Papa Smurf and Lil Man, recently celebrated their ninth birthdays. Fraternal twins, the boys now attend separate schools with one in in-district and the other placed in an out-of-district specialized placement. Kendra believes the separation has been good for the boys, as it has allowed them to develop their own personalities.

Beverly Hughes reports that Marvelous is now age 17 and 6 ft. 4 in. She remains frustrated with Marvelous's service coordination and classroom placement, noting continued difficulties with school district officials. She is looking forward to retiring in 5 years, as she will then spend her days with Marvelous. Post-retirement, she believes Marvelous's need for services will be decreased because she intends to stand in the gap. Beverly plans on spending her days traveling with Marvelous.

As reported in the introduction to participants, **Sarah Mitchell** returned to school to earn a master's degree in special education. She is happy to report that she just recently accepted a position as a full-time special education teacher. The degree and career move were inspired by her son Dwayne. Sarah shared that Dwayne continues to struggle socially and emotionally. As a result, she and her husband are currently pursuing alternative schooling arrangements for him, reviewing in- and out-of-district placements. Sarah believes that while there are many schools out there, they have not found a school with a balance between social-emotional and academic enrichment.

Faith Murphy shared exciting news that she and her husband are expanding their family. They are preparing Fat Daddy for his new role as big brother. Faith and her husband continue to advocate regularly for Fat Daddy, as just recently his third-grade classroom teachers and administrators made overtures to place him in a more restrictive setting. Given her district role as a behavioral therapist, Faith became greatly concerned about the long-term implications of a nonacademic track placement. For now, he remains in the same classroom and will be pushed into general education math and physical education classes. Faith also reports that Fat Daddy now has a service coordinator who will pursue connecting him with community-based social groups and recreational activities. The family just recently placed Fat Daddy on medication to assist with ADHD. Despite initial misgivings about medicine therapy, Faith reported that he is doing well.

Michelle Priest joined my church last year and quickly established herself as "the autism lady," with members now approaching her for assistance on autism-related matters, including community resources, advocacy, and school-related services. Sam accompanies her to church, stands, claps in response to music, and watches his mother sing on the praise team. Michelle continues to expand her autism advocacy by organizing focus groups of Black autism parents. This information will then be shared with an organization seeking to improve services to Black and Latino autism families.

Lisa Thompson emailed updates on John, now age 17. Lisa reports that John is doing well, although still experiencing behavioral issues. The family was able to address some of his behaviors with behavioral therapy, but his clinic case was dropped due to staffing cuts at the agency. She is in the process of getting him reinstated at the clinic, as the therapy previously proved beneficial. John has a new care coordinator and finally received the after-school program placement for which he was long wait-listed. He participates in other respite activities, providing Lisa intervals for self-care and errands. Lisa has begun the process of gaining guardianship of John when he turns 18.

Kiara Williams responded to the call for updates with information about Johnathan's schooling. She shared that she moved him from the public school district to a private Christian academy. Kiara reported that classes are much smaller, and he requires very little in the way of services, receiving only 30 minutes of 1:1 writing support per day. She also mentioned that he received all As and Bs on his last progress report. The opportunity to attend the school was, as she believes, God making a way for Johnathan.

Jeannine Dingus-Eason completed the guardianship process for Caleb, now that he is 19. Shortly after his high school graduation, Caleb moved into an adult group home closer to the city. His level of independence has gradually increased, and he takes pride in organizing family visits and community outings on his own. Caleb attends a day treatment program where he focuses on social skills and job training. He recently decided to apply to a postsecondary program at a local college with autism supports and completed the application on his own. He was accepted and will begin classes soon. Caleb is also looking forward to supported job opportunities on campus. Overall, he is happy, thriving, and continues to tell great jokes. I am proud of him. I am Caleb's mom.

References

Abdullah, M. (2012). Womanist mothering: Loving and raising the revolution. *Western Journal of Black Studies, 36*(1), 57–67.

Abrams, J. A., Maxwell, M., Pope, M., & Belgrave, F. Z. (2014). Carrying the world with the grace of a lady and the grit of a warrior: Deepening our understanding of the "strong Black woman" schema. *Psychology of Women Quarterly, 38*(4), 503–518.

Alexander, M. (2010). *The new Jim Crow: Mass incarceration in the age of colorblindness*. The New Press.

Allen, Q. (2016). "Tell your own story": Manhood, masculinity and racial socialization among Black fathers and their sons. *Ethnic and Racial Studies, 39*(10), 1831–1848. https://doi.org/10.1080/01419870.2015.1110608

Allen, Q., & White-Smith, K. (2018). "That's why I say stay in school": Black mothers' parental involvement, cultural wealth, and exclusion in their son's schooling. *Urban Education, 53*(3), 409–435.

Alston, R. J., & Turner, W. L. (1994). A family strengths model of adjustment to disability for African American clients. *Journal of Counseling & Development, 72*(4), 378–383. https://doi.org/10.1002/j.1556-6676.1994.tb00953.x

Anderson, C., Law, K., Daniels, A., Rice, C., Mandell, D. S., Hagopian, L., & Law, P. (2012). Occurrence and family impact of elopement in children with autism spectrum disorders. *Pediatrics, 130*(5), 1–8.

Angell, A. M., & Solomon, O. (2017). "If I was a different ethnicity, would she treat me the same?" Latino parents' experiences obtaining autism services. *Disability & Society, 32*(8), 1142–1164.

Annamma, S. A., Connor, D., & Ferri, B. (2013). Dis/ability critical race studies (DisCrit): Theorizing at the intersections of race and dis/ability. *Race Ethnicity and Education, 16*(1), 1–31. https://doi.org/10.1080/13613324.2012.730511

Artiles, A. J., Harry, B., Reschly, D. J., & Chinn, P. C. (2002). Over-identification of students of color in special education: A critical overview. *Multicultural Perspectives, 4*(1), 3–10. https://doi.org/10.1207/S15327892MCP0401_2

Avent Harris, J. R. (2019). The Black superwoman in spiritual bypass: Black women's use of religious coping and implications for mental health professionals. *Journal of Spirituality in Mental Health, 23*(2), 180–196.

Avent Harris, J., McKinney, J., & Fripp, J. (2019). "God is a keeper": A phenomenological investigation of Christian African American women's experiences with religious coping. *Professional Counselor, 9*(3), 171–184.

Baio, J., Wiggins, L., Christensen, D. L., Maenner, M. J., Daniels, J., Warren, Z., Kurzius-Spencer, M., Zahorodny, W., Robinson Rosenberg, C., White, T., Durkin, M. S., Imm, P., Nikolaou, L., Yeargin-Allsopp, M., Lee, L., Harrington, R., Lopez, M., Fitzgerald, R. T., Hewitt, A., . . . Dowling, N. (2018). Prevalence of autism spectrum disorder among children aged 8 years—autism and developmental disabilities monitoring network, 11 sites, United States, 2014. *Morbidity and Mortality Weekly Report, 67*(SS-6), 1–23. https://doi.org/10.15585/mmwr.ss6706a1

Baldwin, J. (1993). *The fire next time*. Vintage International.

Barnes, R. J. D. (2016). She was a twin: Black strategic mothering race-work and the politics of survival. *Transforming Anthropology, 24*(1), 49–60.

Bayat, M. (2007). Evidence of resilience in families of children with autism. *Journal of Intellectual Disability Research, 51*(9), 702–714. https://doi.org/10.1111/j.1365-2788.2007.00960

Betancourt, J., Green, A., Carrillo, E., & Aneneh-Firempong, O. (2003). Defining cultural competence: A practical framework for addressing racial/ethnic disparities in health and health care. *Public Health Reports, 118*, 293–302. https://doi.org/10.1093/phr/118.4.293

Bettelheim, B. (1959). Joey: A mechanical boy. *Scientific American, 200*(3), 116–120. https://doi.org/10.1038/SCIENTIFICAMERICAN0359-116

Bettelheim, B. (1967). *The empty fortress: Infantile autism and the birth of the self*. The Free Press.

Botha, M., Dibb, B., & Frost, D. M. (2020). "Autism is me": An investigation of how autistic individuals make sense of autism and stigma. *Disability & Society, 37*(3), 427–453. https://doi.org/10.1080/09687599.2020.1822782

Botha, M., Hanlon, J., & Williams, G. L. (2021). Does language matter? Identity-first versus person-first language use in autism research: A response to Vivanti. *Journal of Autism & Developmental Disorders*. https://doi.org/10.1007/s10803-020-04858-w

Boyd, M., Iacono, I., & McDonald, R. (2019). The perceptions of fathers about parenting a child with developmental disability: A scoping review. *Journal of Policy and Practice in Intellectual Disabilities, 16*(4), 312–324.

Boyd-Franklin, N. (2003). *Black families in therapy: Understanding the African American experience* (2nd ed.). Guilford Press.

Boyd-Franklin, N., & Franklin, A. J. (2000). *Boys into men: Raising our African American teenage boys*. Penguin Putnam.

Broder-Fingert, S., Mateo, C., & Zuckerman, K. E. (2020). Structural racism and autism. *Pediatrics*, *146*(3). https://doi.org/10.1542/peds.2020-015420

Brown, J. R., & Rogers, S. J. (2003). Cultural issues in autism. In J. R. Brown & S. J. Rogers (Eds.), *Autism spectrum disorders: A research review for practitioners* (pp. 209–226). American Psychological Association.

Bryant-Davis, T., & Ocampo, C. (2005). Racist incident-based trauma. *Counseling Psychologist*, *33*, 479–500.

Burkett, K., Morris, E., Anthony, J., Shambley-Ebron, D., & Manning-Courtney, P. (2016). Parenting African American children with autism: The influence of respect and faith in mother, father, single-, and two-parent care. *Journal of Transcultural Nursing*, *28*(5), 496–504. https://doi.org/10.1177/1043659616662316

Burkett, K., Morris, E., Manning-Courtney, P., Anthony, J., & Shambley-Ebron, D. (2015). African American families on autism diagnosis and treatment: The influence of culture. *Journal of Autism and Developmental Disorders*, *45*(10), 3244–3254.

Bush, L. (1999). Am I a man? A literature review engaging the sociohistorical dynamics of Black manhood in the United States. *Western Journal of Black Studies*, *23*(1), 49.

Bush, L. (2000a). Solve for X: Black mothers + Black boys = X. *Journal of African American Men*, *5*(2), 31–53.

Bush, L. (2000b). Black mothers/Black sons: A critical examination of the social science literature. *Western Journal of Black Studies*, *24*(3), 145–155.

Bush, L. (2004). How Black mothers participate in the development of manhood and masculinity: What do we know about Black mothers and their sons? *Journal of Negro Education*, *73*(4), 381–391.

Cabrera, N. J., Ryan, R. M., Mitchell, S. J., Shannon, J. D., & Tamis-LeMonda, C. S. (2008). Low-income, nonresident father involvement with their toddlers: Variation by fathers' race and ethnicity. *Journal of Family Psychology*, *22*(4), 643–647. https://doi.org/10.1037/0893-3200.22.3.643

Carastathis, A. (2014). The concept of intersectionality in feminist theory. *Philosophy Compass*, *9*(5), 304–314.

Carr, T., & Lord, C. (2012). Longitudinal study of perceived negative impact in African American and Caucasian mothers of children with autism spectrum disorder. *Autism*, *17*(4), 405–417. https://doi.org/10.1177/1362361311435155

Cascio, M. A., Weiss, J. A., & Racine, E. (2021). Making autism research inclusive by attending to intersectionality: A review of the research ethics literature. *Review Journal of Autism Development Disorders 8*, 22–36. https://doi.org/10.1007/s40489-020-00204-z

Centers for Disease Control and Prevention. (2020). *Data and statistics on autism spectrum disorder.* http://www.cdc.gov/ncbddd/autism/data.html

Centers for Disease Control and Prevention. (2022, March 31). *Autism and Developmental Disabilities Monitoring (ADDM) Network*. Retrieved September 30, 2022, from https://www.cdc.gov/ncbddd/autism/addm.html

Chapman, T. C., & Bhopal, K. K. (2013). Countering commonsense understandings of "good parenting": Women of color advocating for their children. *Race, Ethnicity and Education, 16*(4), 562–586. https://doi.org/10.1080/13613324.2013.817773

Chivers Yochim, E., & Silva, V. T. (2013). Everyday expertise, autism and "good" mothering in the media discourse of Jenny McCarthy. *Communication and Critical/Cultural Studies, 10*(4), 406–426. https://doi.org/10.1080/14791420.2013.841320

Clark, L. (2014). A humanizing gaze for transcultural nursing research will tell the story of health disparities. *Journal of Transcultural Nursing, 25*(2), 122–128.

Clarke, E. B., McCauley, J. B., & Lord, C. L. (2021). Post-high school daily living skills in autism spectrum disorder. *Journal of the American Academy of Child & Adolescent Psychiatry, 60*(8), 978–985.

Collins, P. H. (1986). Learning from the outsider within: The sociological significance of Black feminist thought. *Social Problems, 33*(6), s14–s32.

Collins, P. H. (1994). Shifting the center: Race, class, and feminist theorizing about motherhood. In D. Bassin, M. Honey & M. M. Kaplan (Eds.), *Representations of motherhood* (pp. 56–74). Yale University Press.

Collins, P. H. (2000). *Black feminist thought: Knowledge, consciousness, and the politics of empowerment* (2nd ed). Routledge.

Collins, P. H. (2016). Shifting the center: Race, class, and feminist theorizing about motherhood. In E. Nakano Glenn, G. Chang, & L. Rennie Forcey (Eds.), *Mothering: Ideology, experience, and agency* (2nd ed., pp. 45–65). Routledge.

Collins, P. H., & Bilge, S. (2016). *Intersectionality*. Polity.

Combahee River Collective. (1982). A Black feminist statement. In G. T. Hull, P. Bell-Scott, & B. Smith (Eds.), *All the women are White, all the Blacks are men, but some of us are brave: Black women's studies* (pp. 13–22). Feminist Press.

Connors, J. L., & Donnellan, A. M. (1998). Walk in beauty: Western perspectives on disability and Navajo family/cultural resilience. In H. I. McCubbin, E. A. Thompson, A. I. Thompson, & J. E. Fromer (Eds.), *Resiliency in Native American and immigrant families* (pp. 159–182). Sage.

Constantino, J. N., Abbacchi, A. M., Saulnier, C., Klaiman, C., Mandell, D. S., Zhang, Y., Hawks, Z., Bates, J., Klin, A., Shattuck, P., Molholm, S., Fitzgerald, R., Roux, A., Lowe, J. K., & Geschwind, D. H. (2020). Timing of the diagnosis of autism in African American children. *Pediatrics, 146*(3). https://doi.org/10.1542/peds.2019-3629

Cooper, C. W., & Christie, C. A. (2005). Evaluating parent empowerment: A look at the potential of social justice evaluation in education. *Teachers College Record, 107*(10), 2248–2271.

Corbin, N. A., Smith, W. A., & Garcia, J. R. (2018). Trapped between justified anger and being the strong Black woman: Black college women coping with racial battle fatigue at historically and predominantly White institutions. *International Journal of Qualitative Studies in Education, 31*(7), 626–643. https://doi.org/10.1080/09518398.2018.1468045

Crenshaw, K. (1991). Race, gender, and sexual harassment. *Southern California Law Review, 65*, 1467–1476.

Cuccaro, M. L., Brinkley, J., Abramson, R. K, Hall, A., Wright, H. H., Hussman, J. P., Gilbert, J. R., & Pericak-Vance, M. A. (2007). Autism in African American families: Clinical-phenotypic findings. *American Journal of Medical Genetics, Part B, 144B*, 1022–1026.

Dancy, T. E., III. (2014). The adultification of Black boys: What educational settings can learn from Trayvon Martin. In K. J. Fasching-Varner, R. E. Reynolds, K. A. Albert, & L. L. Martin (Eds.), *Trayvon Martin, race, and American justice: Teaching race and ethnicity* (pp. 49–55). Sense Publishers.

Davis, A., & Gentlewarrior, S. (2015). White privilege and clinical social work practice: Reflections and recommendations. *Journal of Progressive Human Services, 26*(3), 191–208.

Davis, S. M. (2018). Taking back the power: An analysis of Black women's communicative resistance. *Review of Communication, 18*(4), 301–318. https://oi.org/10.1080/15358593.2018.1461234

Debbaudt, D. (2002). *Autism, advocates, and law enforcement professionals: Recognizing and reducing risk situations for people with autism spectrum disorders*. Jessica Kingsley.

DeGruy, J. (2005). *Post traumatic slave syndrome: America's legacy of enduring injury and healing*. Upton Press.

Delgado Rivera, B., & Rogers-Atkinson, D. (1997). Culturally sensitive interventions: Social skills training with children and parents from culturally and linguistically diverse backgrounds. *Intervention in School and Clinic, 33*(2), 75–80.

DeWolfe, J. (2015). *Parents of children with autism: An ethnography*. Palgrave Macmillan.

DiAngelo, R. (2018). *White fragility: Why it's so hard for White people to talk about racism*. Beacon Press.

DiAquoi, R. (2017). Symbols in the strange fruit seeds: What "the talk" Black parents have with their sons tells us about racism. *Harvard Educational Review, 87*(4), 512–537.

Dixson, A. D., Buras, K. L., & Jeffers, E. K. (2015). The color of reform: Race, education reform, and charter schools in post-Katrina New Orleans. *Qualitative Inquiry, 21*(3), 288–299.

Dottolo, A. L., & Stewart, A. J. (2008). "Don't ever forget now, you're a Black man in America": Intersections of race, class and gender in encounters with the police. *Sex Roles, 59*(5–6), 350–364.

Douglas, P. N. (2013). As if you have a choice: Autism mothers and the remaking of the human. *Health, Culture and Society, 5*(1), 167–181.

Douglas, P. N. (2014). Refrigerator mothers. *Journal of the Motherhood Initiative for Research and Community Involvement, 5*(1), 94–114.

Dow, D. M. (2016). The deadly challenges of raising African American boys: Navigating the controlling image of the "thug." *Gender and Society, 30*(2), 161–188.

Ducharme, L. J., Knudsen, H. K., & Roman, P. M. (2007). Emotional exhaustion and turnover intention in human service occupations: The protective role of coworker support. *Sociological Spectrum, 28*, 81–104.

Dudley, K. M., Klinger, M. R., Meyer, A., Powell, P., & Klinger, L. G. (2019). Understanding service usage and needs for adults with ASD: The importance of living situation. *Journal of Autism and Developmental Disorders, 49*, 556–568. https://doi.org/10.1007/s10803-018-3729-0

Duerte, C. S., Bordin, I. A., Yazigi, L., & Mooney, J. (2005). Factors associated with stress in mothers of children with autism. *Autism, 9*(4), 416–427.

Dumas, M. J., & Nelson, J. D. (2016). (Re)Imagining Black boyhood: Toward a critical framework for educational research. *Harvard Educational Review, 86*(1), 27–47.

Dunn, M. E., Burbine, T., Bowers, C. A., & Tantleff-Dunn, S. (2001). Moderators of stress in parents of children with autism. *Community Mental Health Journal, 37*(1), 39–52.

Durkin, M. S., Maenner, M. J., Baio, J., Christensen, D., Daniels, J., Fitzgerald, R., Imm, P., Lee, L., Schieve, L. A., Van Naarden Braun, K., Wingate, M. A., & Yeargin-Allsopp, M. (2017). Autism spectrum disorder among US children (2002-2010): Socioeconomic, racial, and ethnic disparities. *American Journal of Public Health, 107*(11), 1818–1826.

Dyches, T. T., Wilder, L. K., Sudweeks, R. R., Obiakor, F. E., & Algozzine, B. (2004). Multicultural issues in autism. *Journal of Autism and Developmental Disorders, 34*(2) 211–222.

Eilenberg, J. S., Paff, M., Harrison, A. J., & Long, K. A. (2019). Disparities based on race, ethnicity, and socioeconomic status over the transition to adulthood among adolescents and young adults on the autism spectrum: A systematic review. *Current Psychiatry Reports, 21*(5), 1–16. https://doi.org/10.1007/s11920-019-1016-1

Elder, J. (2013). Empowering families in the treatment of autism. In M. Fitzgerald (Ed.), *Recent advances in autism spectrum disorders, vol. I*. IntechOpen.

Ennis-Cole, D., Durodoye, B. A., & Harris, H. L. (2013). The impact of culture on autism diagnosis and treatment: Considerations for counselors and other professionals. *Family Journal: Counseling and Therapy for Couples and Families, 21*(3), 279–287. https://doi.org/10.1177/1066480713476834

Eyal, G., & Hart, B. (2010). How parents of autistic children became "experts on their own children": Notes towards a sociology of expertise. *Berkeley Journal of Sociology*, *54*, 3–17. https://doi.org/10.2307/40999932

Fish, W. (2006). Perceptions of parents of students with autism towards the IEP meeting: A case study of one family support group chapter. *Education*, *127*(1), 56–68.

Fish, W. (2009). Educator perceptions toward the IEP Meeting. *Academic Leadership: The Online Journal*, *7*(4), Article 12. https://scholars.fhsu.edu/alj/vol7/iss4/12

Gantt, A. L., & Greif, G. L. (2009). African American single mothers raising sons: Implications for family therapy. *Journal of Family Social Work*, *12*(3), 227–243. https://doi.org/10.1080/10522150903030014

Gardner, L., Campbell, J. M., & Westdal, J. (2019). Brief report: Descriptive analysis of law enforcement officers' experiences with and knowledge of autism. *Journal of Autism and Development Disorders*, *49*, 1278–1283. https://doi.org/10.1007/s10803-018-3794-4

Gay, G. (2010). *Culturally responsive teaching: Theory, research, and practice*. Teachers College Press.

Goff, P., Jackson, M., & Di Leone, B. (2014). The essence of innocence: Consequences of dehumanizing Black children. *Journal of Personality and Social Psychology*, *106*(4), 526–545.

Goin-Kochel, R. P., Mackintosh, V. H., & Myers, B. J. (2006). How many doctors does it take to make an autism spectrum diagnosis? *Autism*, *10*(5), 439–451.

Gourdine, R. M., Bafflour, T. D., & Teasley, M. (2011). Autism and the African American community. *Social Work in Public Health*, *26*(4). https://doi.org/10.1080/19371918.2011.579499

Green, K. M., Ensminger, M. E., Robertson, J. A., & Juon, H. (2006). Impact of adult sons' incarceration on African American mothers' psychological distress. *Journal of Marriage and Family*, *68*(2), 430–441.

Hannon, M. D., & Hannon, L. V. (2017). Fathers' orientation to their children's autism diagnosis: A grounded theory study. *Journal of Autism and Developmental Disorders*, *47*(7), 2265–2274. https://doi.org/10.1007/s10803-017-3149-6

Hannon, M., White, E., & Nadrich, T. (2018). Influence of autism on fathering style among Black fathers: A narrative inquiry. *Journal of Family Therapy*, *40*, 224–246.

Harry, B. (2007). Collaboration with culturally and linguistically diverse families: Ideal versus reality. *Exceptional Children*, *74*(3), 372–388. https://doi.org/10.1177/001440290807400306

Harry, B., Klingner, J. K., & Hart, J. (2005). African American families under fire: Ethnographic views of family strengths. *Remedial and Special Education*, *26*(2), 101–112.

Heitzeg, N. A. (2016). *The school-to-prison pipeline: Education, discipline, and racialized double standards*. Praeger.

Hendricks, D. R., & Wehman, P. (2009). Transition from school to adulthood for youth with autism spectrum disorders. *Focus on Autism and Other Developmental Disabilities, 24*(2), 77–88. https://doi.org/10.1177/1088357608329827

Hill, S. A. (2001). Class, race, and gender dimensions of child rearing in African American families. *Journal of Black Studies, 31*(4), 494–508.

Hilton, C. L., Fitzgerald, R. T., Jackson, K. M., Maxim, R. A., Bosworth, C. C., Shattuck, P. T., Geschwind, D. H., & Constantino, J. N. (2010). Brief report: Under-representation of African Americans in autism genetic research: A rationale for inclusion of subjects representing diverse family structures. *Journal of Autism Developmental Disorders, 40*, 633–639. https://doi.org/10.1007/s10803-009-0905-2

Houston, M. (2000). Multiple perspectives: African American women conceive their talk. *Women and Language, 1*(23), 11–17.

Jacobs, L., Lawlor, M., & Mattingly, C. (2011). I/We narratives among African American families raising children with special needs. *Culture, Medicine, and Psychiatry, 35*, 3–25. https://doi.org/10.1007/s11013-010-9196-5

Jones, D. R., & Mandell, D. S. (2020). To address racial disparities in autism research, we must think globally, act locally. *Autism, 24*(7), 1587–1589. https://doi.org/10.1177/1362361320948313

Jones, L. V., Mountz, S. E., Trant, J., & Quezada, N. M. (2019). A Black feminist approach for caseworkers intervening with Black female caregivers. *Journal of Public Child Welfare, 14*(4), 395–411. https://doi.org/10.1080/15548732.2019.1621234

Kalyanpur, M., Harry, B., & Skrtic, T. (2000). Equity and advocacy expectations of culturally diverse families' participation in special education. *International Journal of Disability, Development and Education, 47*(2), 119–136.

Kanner, L. (1943). Autistic disturbances of affective contact. *Nervous Child, 2*, 217–250.

King, J., & Mitchell, C. (1995). *Black mothers to sons: Juxtaposing African American literature with social practice (counterpoints)*. Peter Lang.

King, S. V. (1998). The beam in thine own eye: Disability and the Black church. *Western Journal of Black Studies, 22*(1), 37.

King, S. V. (2001). "God won't put more on you than you can bear": Faith as a coping strategy among older African American caregiving parents of adult children with disabilities. *Journal of Religion, Disability & Health, 4*, 7–24. https://doi.org/10.1300/JO95v04n04_02

King, S. V. (2002). The intracultural crippling of African Americans with disabilities. In J. L. Conyers (Ed.), *Black culture and race relations* (pp. 293–310). Rowman & Littlefield.

King, V., Harris, K., & Heard, H. (2004). Racial and ethnic diversity in nonresident father involvement. *Journal of Marriage and Family*, *66*(1), 1–21. http://www.jstor.org/stable/3599862

Kirby, A. V. (2016). Parent expectations mediate outcomes for young adults with autism spectrum disorder. *Journal of Autism and Developmental Disorders*, *46*(5), 1643–55.

Kolomer, S., McCallion, P., & Janicki, M. P. (2002). African-American grandmother carers of children with disabilities: Preliminary comparisons. *Journal of Gerontological Social Work*, *33*, 45–63.

Kübler-Ross, E. (1973). *On death and dying: What the dying have to teach doctors, nurses, clergy and their own families*. Routledge.

Kunjufu, J. (1985). *Countering the conspiracy to destroy Black boys, vol. 1*. African American Images.

Ladson-Billings, G. (1995). Toward a theory of culturally relevant pedagogy. *American Educational Research Journal*, *32*(3), 465–491.

Ladson-Billings, G. (2011). Boyz to men? Teaching to restore Black boys' childhood. *Race Ethnicity and Education*, *14*(1), 7–15. https://doi.org/10.1080/13613324.2011.531977

Langan, M. (2011). Parental voices and controversies in autism. *Disability & Society*, *26*(2), 193–205. https://doi.org/10.1080/09687599.2011.544059

Lareau, A., & Horvat, E. M. (1999). Moments of social inclusion and exclusion: Race, class and cultural capital in family-school relationships. *Sociology of Education*, *72*(1), 37–53.

Lei, J., Jones, L., & Brosnan, M. (2021). Exploring an e-learning community's response to the language and terminology use in autism from two massive open online courses on autism education and technology use. *Autism*, *25*(5), 1349–1367. https://doi.org/10.1177/1362361320987963

Leininger, M. (1991). Becoming aware of types of health practitioners and cultural imposition. *Journal of Transcultural Nursing*, *2*(2), 32–39. https://doi.org/10.1177/104365969100200205

Leininger, M. M., & McFarland, M. R. (Eds.) (2006). *Culture diversity & universality: A worldwide nursing theory* (2nd ed.). Jones and Bartlett.

Lobar, S. L. (2014). Family adjustments across cultural groups in autism spectrum disorders. *Advances in Nursing Science*, *37*(2), 174–186.

Lopez, K. (2014). Sociocultural perspectives of Latino children with autism spectrum disorder. *Best Practices in Mental Health*, *10*(2), 15–31.

Lopez, K., Xu, Y., Magana, S., & Guzman, J. (2018). Mothers' reaction to autism diagnosis: A qualitative analysis comparing Latino and White parents. *Journal of Rehabilitation*, *84*(1), 41–50.

Lovelace, T. S., Comis, M., Tabb, J. M., & Oshokoya, O. E. (2021, June 28). *Missing from the narrative: A seven decade scoping review of the inclusion of Black autistic women and girls in autism research*. https://doi.org/10.31234/osf.io/d3v29

Malone, K. M., Pearson, J. N., Palazzo, K. N., Manns, L. D., Rivera, A. Q., & Mason Martin, D. L. (2022). The scholarly neglect of Black autistic adults in autism research. *Autism in Adulthood*. http://doi.org/10.1089/aut.2021.0086

Mandara, J., Varner, F., & Richman, S. (2010). Do African American mothers really "love" their sons and "raise" their daughters? *Journal of Family Psychology, 24*(1), 41–50.

Mandell, D. S., & Novak, M. (2005). The role of culture in families' treatment decisions for children with autism spectrum disorders. *Mental Retardation and Developmental Disabilities Research Reviews, 11*(2), 110–115. https://doi.org/10.1002/mrdd.20061

Mandell, D. S., & Salzer, M. S. (2007). Who joins support groups among parents of children with autism? *Autism, 11*(2), 111–122. https://doi.org/10.1177/1362361307077506

Mandell, D. S., Wiggins, L. D., Carpenter, L. A., Daniels, J., DiGuiseppi, C., Durkin, M. S., & Kirby, R. S. (2009). Racial/ethnic disparities in the identification of children with autism spectrum disorders. *American Journal of Public Health, 99*(3), 493–498.

Manoucheka, C. (2018). "What now?" The wailing Black women, grief, and difference. *Black Camera, 9*(2), 110–131.

Marchand, A. D., Vasar, R. R., Diemer, M. A., & Rowley, S. (2019). Integrating race, racism and critical consciousness in Black parents' engagement with schools. *Journal of Family Theory & Review, 11*, 367–384. https://doi.org/10.1111/jftr.12344

Marsack, C. N., & Perry, T. E. (2018). Aging in place in every community: Social exclusion experiences of parents of adult children with autism spectrum disorder. *Research on Aging, 40*(6), 535–557. https://doi.org/10.1177/0164027517717044

Marshall, B., Kollia, B., Wagner, V., & Yablonsky, D. (2018). Identifying depression in parents of children with autism spectrum disorder: Recommendations for professional practice. *Journal of Psychosocial Nursing and Mental Health Services, 56*(4), 23–27.

Marvin, R. S., & Pianta, R. C. (1996). Mothers' reactions to their child's diagnosis: Relations with security of attachment. *Journal of Clinical Child Psychology, 25*(4), 436–445.

Mattis, J. S. (2002). Religion and spirituality in the meaning-making and coping experiences of African American women: A qualitative analysis. *Psychology of Women Quarterly, 26*, 309–321.

Maye, M., Boyd, B. A., Martínez-Pedraza, F., Halladay, A., Thurm, A., & Mandell, D. S. (2022). Biases, barriers, and possible solutions: Steps towards addressing autism researchers' under-engagement with racially, ethnically, and socio-

economically diverse communities. *Journal of Autism and Developmental Disorders, 52*(9), 4206–4211.
McDonald, K. B. (1997). Black activist mothering: Historical intersections of race, gender, and class. *Gender in Society, 11*(6), 773–795.
Modell, S. J., & Copp, D. (2007). Police officers and disability: Perceptions and attitudes. *Intellectual and Developmental Disabilities, 45*(1), 60–63.
Moh, T. A., & Magiati, I. (2012). Factors associated with parental stress and satisfaction during the process of diagnosis of children with autism spectrum disorders. *Research in Autism Spectrum Disorders, 6*(1), 293–303.
Montes, G., & Halterman, J. S. (2011). White-Black disparities in family-centered care among children with autism in the United States: Evidence from the NS-CSHCN 2005-2006. *American Pediatrics, 11*, 297–304.
Morgan, E. H., & Stahmer, A. C. (2020). Narratives of single, Black mothers using cultural capital to access autism interventions in schools. *British Journal of Sociology of Education, 42*(1), 48–65.
Morris, J. K. (1992). Personal power in Black mothers of handicapped sons. *Affilia, 7*(3), 72–92.
Myers, B. J., Mackintosh, V. H., & Goin-Kochel, R. P. (2009). "My greatest joy and my greatest heart ache": Parents' own words on how having a child in the autism spectrum has affected their lives and their families' lives. *Research in Autism Spectrum Disorders, 3*(3) 670–684. https://doi.org/10.1016/j.rasd.2009.01.004
National Association for the Advancement of Colored People (NAACP). (2016). *Criminal justice fact sheet.* http://www.naacp.org/pages/criminal-justice-fact-sheet
National Autistic Society. (2011). *Autism: A guide for criminal justice professionals.* http://www.autism.org.uk/products/core-nas-publications/autism-a-guide-for-criminal-justice-professionals.aspx
Nickerson, K. J., Helms, J. E., & Terrell, F. (1994). Cultural mistrust, opinions about mental illness, and Black students' attitudes toward seeking psychological help from White counselors. *Journal of Counseling Psychology, 41*(3), 378–385.
Noguera, P. (2008). *The trouble with Black boys: And other reflections on race, equity, and the future of public education.* Jossey-Bass.
Okundaye, J. (2021, May 27). Ask a self-advocate: The pros and cons of person-first and identity-first language. Massachusetts Advocates for Children. https://www.massadvocates.org/news/ask-a-self-advocate-the-pros-and-cons-of-person-first-and-identity-first-language
Osborn, L. A., & Reed, P. (2008). Parents' perceptions of communication with professionals during the diagnosis of autism. *Autism, 12*(3), 309–324.
Pearson, J. N., & Meadan, H. (2021). FACES: An advocacy intervention for African American parents of children with autism. *Intellectual and Developmental Disabilities, 59*(2), 155–171.

Pierce, N. P., O'Reilly, M. F., Sorrells, A. M., Fragale, C. L. White, P. J., Aguilar, J. M., & Cole, H. A. (2014). Ethnicity reporting practices for empirical research in autism-related journals. *Journal of Autism and Developmental Disorders*, *44*(7), 1507–1519.

Priester, M., Pitner, R., & Lackey, R. (2017). Examining the relationship between diversity exposure and students' color-blind racial attitudes and awareness of racial oppression. *Journal of Ethnic & Cultural Diversity in Social Work*, *28*(2), 229–245. https://doi.org/10.1080/15313204.2017.1344948

Pruchno, R., Patrick, J. H., & Burant, C. J. (1997). African American and White mothers of adults with chronic disabilities: Caregiving burden and satisfaction. *Family Relations*, *46*(4), 335–346. https://doi.org/10.149.69.232.79

Reed, T. D., & Neville, H. A. (2014). The influence of religiosity and spirituality on psychological well-being among Black women. *Journal of Black Psychology*, *40*(4), 384–401. https://doi.org/10.1177/0095798413490956

Richie, B. E. (1999). The social construction of the "immoral" Black mother: Social policy, community policing, and effects on youth violence. In A. E. Clarke & V. L. Olesen (Eds.), *Revisioning women, health, and healing* (pp. 283–299). Routledge.

Rodas, J. M. (2021). Black autism: A conversation with Diana Paulin. *College Language Association*, *64*(1), 121–126.

Rogers, A. (2015). How police brutality harms mothers: Linking police violence to the reproductive justice movement. *Hastings Race & Poverty Law Journal*, *12*(2), 205–232.

Rogers-Dulan, J., & Blacher, J. (1995). African American families, religion, and disability: A conceptual framework. *Mental Retardation*, *33*(4), 226–238.

Rose, A. (1997). "Who causes the blind to see": Disability and quality of religious life. *Disability and Society*, *12*(3), 395–405.

Roux, A. M., Rast, J. E., Garfield, T., Shattuck, P., & Shea, L. L. (2021). *National autism indicators report: Family perspectives on services and supports*. Life Course Outcomes Research Program, A. J. Drexel Autism Institute, Drexel University. https://drexel.edu/autismoutcomes/publications-and-reports/publications/nair-family-perspectives-on-services-and-supports/

Roux, A. M., Shattuck, P. T., Rast, J. E., Rava, J. A., & Anderson, K. A. (2015). *National autism indicators report: Transition into young adulthood*. Life Course Outcomes Research Program, A. J. Drexel Autism Institute, Drexel University. https://drexel.edu/autismoutcomes/publications-and-reports/publications/National-Autism-Indicators-Report-Transition-to-Adulthood/

Rowley, S. J., Helaire, L. J., & Banerjee, M. (2010). Reflecting on racism: School involvement and perceived teacher discrimination in African American mothers. *Journal of Applied Developmental Psychology*, *31*(1), 83–92.

Saldana, J. (2016). *The coding manual for qualitative researchers* (3rd ed.). Sage.

Seltzer, M. M., Wyngaarden, K., Shattuck, P. T., Orsmond, G., Swe, A., & Lord, C. (2003). The symptoms of autism spectrum disorders in adolescence and adulthood. *Journal of Autism and Developmental Disorders, 33*(6), 565–581.

Shaia, W. E., Nichols, H. M., Dababnah, S., Campion, K., & Garbino, N. (2020). Brief report: Participation of Black and African-American families in autism research. *Journal of Autism and Developmental Disorders, 50*, 1841–1846. https://doi.org/10.1007/s10803-019-03926-0

Shattuck, P. T., Narendorf, S. C., Cooper, B., Sterzing, P. R., Wagner, M., & Taylor, J. L. (2012). Postsecondary education and employment among youth with an autism spectrum disorder. *Pediatrics, 129*(6), 1042. https://doi.org/10.1542/peds.2011-2864

Siller, M., Morgan, L., Swanson, M., & Hotez, E. (2013). Promoting early identification of autism in the primary care setting: Bridging the gap between what we know and what we do. In M. Fitzgerald (Ed.), *Recent advances in autism spectrum disorders, vol. I*. IntechOpen.

Siller, M., Reyes, N., Hotez, E., Hutman, T., & Sigman, M. (2013). Longitudinal change in the use of services in autism spectrum disorder: Understanding the role of child characteristics, family demographics, and parent cognitions. *Autism, 18*(4), 1–14.

Simpson, D. E. (2003). *Refrigerator mothers*. Kartemquin Films.

Sivberg, B. (2002). Family system and coping behaviors: A comparison between parents of children with autistic spectrum disorders and parents with non-autistic children. *Autism, 6*(4), 397–409.

Smith, P. (2020, May 14). Chicago is set to pay $2.25 million for shooting of Ricardo Hayes. WBEZ Chicago. https://www.wbez.org/stories/chicago-set-to-pay-225m-for-unjustified-shooting-of-unarmed-teen-with-disabilities/542c204a-de40-4bf6-8328-a350eef576d2

Smitherman, G. (1986). *Talkin' and testifying: The language of Black America*. Wayne State University Press.

Solomon, O., & Lawlor, M. C. (2013). "And I look down and he is gone": Narrating autism, elopement and wandering in Los Angeles. *Social Science & Medicine, 94*, 106–114. https://doi.org/10.1016/j.socscimed.2013.06.034

Sousa, A. C. (2015). "Crying doesn't work": Emotion and parental involvement of working class mothers raising children with developmental disabilities. *Disability Studies Quarterly, 35*(1), 1–6. https://doi.org/10.18061/dsq.v35i1.3966

Spano, R., Rivera, C., & Bolland, J. M. (2011). Does parenting shield youth from exposure to violence during adolescence? A 5-year longitudinal test in a high-poverty sample of minority youth. *Journal of Interpersonal Violence, 26*(5), 930–949. https://doi.org/10.1177/0886260510365873

Stack, C. B. (1974). *All our kin: Strategies for survival in a Black community*. Harper & Row.

Stack, C. B., & Burton, L. M. (2016). Kinscripts: Reflections on family, generation, and culture. In E. Nakano Glenn, G. Chang, & L. Rennie Forcey (Eds.), *Mothering: Ideology, experience, and agency* (2nd ed., pp. 33–43). Routledge.

Stahmer, A. C., Vejnoska, S., Iadarola, S., Straiton, D., Segovia, F. R., Luelmo, P., Morgan, E. H., Lee, H. S., Javed, A., Bronstein, B., Hochheimer, A., Cho, E., Aranbarri, A., Mandell, D., Hassrick, E. M., Smith, T., & Kasari, C. (2019). Caregiver voices: Cross-cultural input on improving access to autism services. *Journal of Racial and Ethnic Health Disparities, 6*(4), 752–773.

Stanley, S. L. G. (2015). The advocacy efforts of African American mothers of children with disabilities in rural special education: Considerations for school professionals. *Rural Special Education Quarterly, 34*(4), 3–17.

Steinbrenner, J. R., McIntyre, N., Rentschler, L. F., Pearson, J. N., Luelmo, P., Jaramillo, M. E., & Hume, K. A. (2022). Patterns in reporting and participant inclusion related to race and ethnicity in autism intervention literature: Data from a large-scale systematic review of evidence-based practices. *Autism, 26*(8), 2026–2040. https://doi.org/10.1177/13623613211072

Stoner, J. B., Jones Bock, S., Thompson, J. R., Angell, M. E., Heyl, B. S., & Crowley, E. P. (2005). Welcome to our world: Parent perceptions of interactions between parents of young children with ASD and education professionals. *Focus on Autism and Other Developmental Disabilities, 20*(1), 39–51.

Straiton, D., & Sridhar, A. (2022). Call to action for autism clinicians in response to anti-Black racism. *Autism, 26*(4), 988–994.

Tarakeshwar, N., & Pargament, K. I. (2001). Religious coping in families of children with autism. *Focus in Autism and Other Developmental Disabilities, 16*, 247–260.

Taylor, J. L., & Seltzer, M. M. (2011). Employment and post-secondary educational activities for young adults with autism spectrum disorders during the transition to adulthood. *Journal of Autism Developmental Disorders, 41*(5), 566–574. https://doi.org/10.1007/s10803-010-1070-3

Terhune, P. S. (2005). African-American developmental disability discourses: Implications for policy development. *Journal of Policy and Practice in Intellectual Disabilities, 2*, 18–28. https://doi.org/10.1111/j.1741-1130.2005.00004.x

Tincani, M., Travers, J., & Boutout, A. (2009). Race, culture, and autism spectrum disorder: Understanding the role of diversity in successful educational interventions. *Research & Practice for Persons with Severe Disabilities, 34*(3–4), 81–90.

Veness, C., Prior, M., Bavin, E., Eadie, P., Cini, E., & Reilly, S. (2012). Early indicators of autism spectrum disorders at 12 and 24 months of age: A prospective, longitudinal comparative study. *Autism, 16*(2), 163–177.

Vivanti, G. (2020). Ask the editor: What is the most appropriate way to talk about individuals with a diagnosis of autism? *Journal of Autism and Developmental Disorders, 50*(2), 691–693. https://doi.org/10.1007/s10803-019-04280-x

Washington, H. A. (2006). *Medical apartheid: The dark history of medical experimentation on Black Americans from colonial times to the present*. Harlem Moon.

Waters, B. S. (2016). Freedom lessons: Black mothers asserting smartness of their children. *Race Ethnicity and Education, 19*(6), 1223–1235.

Whitaker, T. R., & Snell, C. L. (2016). Parenting while powerless: Consequences of "the talk." *Journal of Human Behavior in the Social Environment, 26*(3–4), 303–309. https://doi.org/10.1080/10911359.2015.1127736.

Wiggins, L. D., Baio, J., & Rice, C. (2006). Examination of the time between first evaluation and first autism spectrum diagnosis in a population-based sample. *Journal of Developmental and Behavioral Pediatrics, 27*(2), S79–S87.

Wilson, G., Dunham, R., & Alpert, G. (2004). Prejudice in police profiling. *American Behavioral Scientist, 47*(7), 896–909. https://doi.org/10.1177/0002764203261069

Wilson Cooper, C. (2007) School choice as 'motherwork': Valuing African-American women's educational advocacy and resistance. *International Journal of Qualitative Studies in Education, 20*(5), 491–512. https://doi.org/10.1080/09518390601176655

Woods-Giscombe, C. (2010). Superwoman schema: African American women's views on stress, strength, and health. *Qualitative Health Research, 20*(5), 668–683.

Woods-Giscombe, C., Allen, A., Black, A., Steed, T., Li, Y., & Lackey, C. (2019) The Giscombe Superwoman Schema Questionnaire: Psychometric Properties and Associations with Mental Health and Health Behaviors in African American Women. *Issues in Mental Health Nursing, 40*(8), 672–681. https://doi.org/10.1080/01612840.2019.1584654

Yancy, G., del Guadalupe Davidson, M., & Hadley, S. (2016). *Our Black sons matter: Mothers talk about fears, sorrows, and hopes*. Rowman & Littlefield.

Yee, A. (2016). Autism research's overlooked racial bias. *The Atlantic*. http://www.theatlantic.com/health/archive/2016/05/autism-research-overlooked-racialbias/481314/

Zionts, L. T., Zionts, P., Harrison, S., & Bellinger, O. (2003). Urban African American families' perceptions of cultural sensitivity within the special education system. *Focus on Autism and Other Developmental Disabilities, 18*(1), 41–50. https://doi.org/10.1177/108835760301800106

Index

acceptance, picture of action, 47–51
adjustments, post-diagnosis actions, 49
adult autism services, 150–51
advocacy
    for autism, 12–13, 37, 116, 119, 170, 192
    class implications of, 103–6
    confronting oppressive systems, 109–16
    and service providers, 180–83
    warrior mother, 13
agencies, expectations for, 142–45
American Sign Language (ASL), 27
Andrew, son with autism, 30, 33, 84, 107, 190
Angell, M. E., 13
applied behavioral analysis (ABA), 101
attention-deficit hyperactivity disorder (ADHD), 22
autism
    BAMs and representation of, 117–45
    in Black churches, 128–32
    Black family perspectives on, 13–16
    coping with, 62–64
    cultural scene, 121–26
    diagnosing, 2
    diagnosis overview, 9–10
    historical representation of autism mothers, 10–12
    intersection. *See* intersection, race-class-gender-autism
    knowledge of, 13, 41, 47, 51–54, 99–103, 119, 128, 175–76, 178, 181
    label of, 51
    search for community, 1, 3
    "the talk," 80–87
    warrior mothers and, 12–13
autism acceptance model. *See* post-diagnosis response
Autism in Black, 118
Autism Mocha Moms, 118
autism spaces, 171
autism spectrum disorder (ASD), 9–10, xv
    Black family perspectives on, 13–16
    children with, 10, 13, 15, 16, 148
    diagnoses, 10, 16, 22, 24, 45, 49
    knowledge, 36–37
    research, 14–15
    young adults with, 15
"Autistic Disturbances of Affective Contact," 10
awareness, police brutality, 76–80

Bear, son with autism, 30–31, 129–30, 159, 161, 189

Betancourt, J., 133
Bettelheim, Bruno, 11
Bhopal, K. K., 96
Bilge, S., 18
Black autism mothers (BAMs), 3–7, 167–70
  and active members of society, 155–58
  autism representation and, 117–45
  building trust with, 99–103
  class implications of advocacy of, 103–6
  creating cultural spaces, 126–28
  and future, 147–65
  interpretation of, 106–9
  intersectional considerations for, 172–75
  involvement with special education, 97–106
  making of, 27–41
  police brutality awareness, 76–80
  post-diagnosis response, 43–68
  race-class-gender-autism intersection, 69–92
  refrigerator mothers and, 10–12
  revisiting conceptualizations of, 170–72
  self-compassion, 64–66
  study participants, 31–41
  "the talk," 80–87
Black boyhood, innocence of, 73–76
Black English Vernacular, 4
Black families, intersectional considerations for, 174–77
Black Lives Matter, 77
Black men, 152–55
  serving as active members of society, 155–58
Black people, 50, 70, 77, 80, 82, 91, 117, 135, 170
  boyhood, 73–76
  family perspectives on autism, 13–16
  mothers and sons, 16–18

Boston, Donelle, participant, 31–32, 80, 129, 135, 155, 159, 161, 189
Boyd, B. A., 54
boyhood, protecting innocence of, 73–76
brutality, police, 76–80
Burkett, K., 16

Caleb, child, xv–xviii, 43–44
Casey Foundation, 16
Cat Man, son with autism, 30, 36, 38, 85, 86, 150
Centers for Disease Control and Prevention (CDC), 9
Chapman, T. C., 96
Charles, Candi, participant, 32
  "I don't want him to be the inheritance . . . ," 158–59
  in Black churches, 130–31, 178
  and class implications, 105–6
  on creating cultural spaces, 126–28
  race-class-gender-autism intersection, 87–91
  raising successful and good Black men, 152–54
  strategizing autism learning cruve, 51–52
Charles, Pappas, incident involving, 87–92
Chavez, Caesar, 119
child rearing, 14, 16, 59, 136, 176
Christian, Marley, participant, 32–33, 49, 51, 61, 63, 131–32, 137, 190
  and autism cultural scene, 122–26
churches
  autism in, 128–32
  international considerations for, 177–80
clinicians, expectations for, 139–42
Collins, P. H., 15, 18, 20
Color of Autism Foundation, 118
Committee on Special Education (CSE), 97–98

community, support from, 59–61
conspiracy, 28–29
constellation. *See* family constellation
Cooper, Wilson, 96
coping, religion as, 62–64
criminalization, Black men, 18
cultural competence
  concept, 132–34
  sociopolitical consciousness, 136–39
cultural scene, 121–26
cultural space
  autism, 119–21
  Black churches, 128–32
  creating, 126–28
  revisiting conceptualizations of mothers, 170–72
culturally competent health care, 133
culturally responsive autism care and services, 132–34
Cuomo, Andrew, 107

Daniels, Karla, participant, 33–34, 83–84, 107–8, 136, 190
Debbaudt, D., 184
DeGruy, J., 137
DiAngelo, R., 91, 171
DisCrit, 183
Douglas, P. N., 11, 19, 120
Dumas, M. J., 73–76
Dwayne, son with autism, 30, 37, 56, 60, 64, 154, 191

early infantile autism, 10–11
Ebony magazine, 117
education, race-class-gender-autism intersection
  BAM interpretation, 106–9
  confronting oppressive systems, 109–16
  overview, 93–97
  special education, 97–106
educators, intersectional considerations for, 180–83

Elder, J., 45
Elijah, son with autism, 30, 34–35, 65, 85, 110–14, 135, 159
Ennis-Cole, D., 151
expectations
  agencies, 142–45
  clinicians, 139–42
  researchers, 139–42
  service care coordinators, 142–45

family constellation, 59–61
Fat Daddy, son with autism, 30, 38, 55, 60–61, 191–92
fathers, helping, 54–59
Floyd, George, 77
Fox, Thelma, participant, 34–35, 75, 84–85, 160, 190
  giving power back, 114–15
  sacrifices for special education services, 110–12
  at school meeting, 113–14
  on sociopolitical consciousness, 135
future, hope for, 147–49
  adult autism services, 150–51
  raising successful and good Black men, 152–58
  sons' independence, 160–65
  studying long-term outcomes, 158–60

Gay, Geneva, 134
Gourdine, R. M., 139
Green, Kendra, participant, 35–36, 53, 122, 125–26, 142–43, 191

Harry, B., 107
Hayes, Ricardo, 77
healing autism house, 131–32
hegemonic notion, 76
Heitzeg, N. A., 73
high stress-low pay nature, 143–44
honesty, importance of, 155–58

Hughes, Beverly, participant, 36, 106–7, 144, 162–63, 191
husbands, helping, 54–59
hyper-referrals, 97
hypersurveillance, 73, 75, 84, 92

inaction, 141–42
independence, studying, 160–65
Individuals with Disabilities Education Act, 117
innocence, protecting, 73–76
intersection, race-class-gender-autism, 69–73
  Black mothers, 69–92
  education, 93–116
  police brutality, 76–80
  protecting innocence, 73–76
  sons' independence, 160–65
  "the talk," 80–87
  true-to-life experience, 87–92
intersectionality, 18–20

Jet magazine, 117
John, son with autism, 30, 40, 57–58, 65, 82–83, 100, 144, 151, 155–56, 160–61, 192
Johnathan, son with autism, 30, 40–41, 61–62, 99, 108, 152, 192
Journal of Autism and Developmental Disorders, 4

Kanner, Leo, 10–11
King, S. V., 14
knowledge, autism, 13, 41, 47, 51–54, 99–103, 119, 128, 175–76, 178, 181
Kunjufu, Jawanza, 17, 28

Lacks, Henrietta, 135
Ladson-Billings, Gloria, 75, 134
Langan, M., 121
law enforcement, intersectional considerations for, 183–85

Lawrence, Ginger, participant, 36–37, 48, 63, 66, 85–86, 137, 178, 189
learning curve, strategizing, 51–54
Lil Man, son with autism, 35, 122, 191
long-term outcomes, studying, 158–60
Lopez, K., 46, 98

Mandela, Nelson, 119
marginalized positionality, 16
Marvelous, son with autism, 30, 36, 162–63, 191
Marvin, R. S., 45–46
Maye, M., 124
McCarthy, Jenny, 13
Meadan, H., 103
middle class, 103–6
Mikey, son with autism, 30, 34, 83–84, 107, 190
Mitchell, Sarah, participant, 30, 37, 55–56, 60, 127–28, 154–55, 191
Mitchell, C., 14
Mocha Autism Network, 118
mothering. *See* Black autism mothers (BAMs)
mothers
  Black mothers and sons, 16–18
  historical representation, 10–12
  refrigerator mothers, 10–12
  revisiting conceptualizations of, 170–72
  self-compassion, 64–66
  warrior mothers, 12–13
motherwork, 18–20
Murphy, Faith, participant, 30, 37–38, 48–50, 55, 60, 63, 78, 104, 108–9, 191–92
Music Man, son with autism, 30, 36, 48, 63, 85, 150

needs, centering, 54–59
Nelson, J. D., 73–76
new normal, creating, 54–59
Newton, Huey P., 119

Noguera, P., 17
normal, descriptor, 79–80

obsessive-compulsive disorder (OCD), xv
occupational therapy (OT), 183
Odum, Indigo, participant, 30, 38–39, 160–61
  acceptance in action, 50–53
  building trust with BAMs, 100–101
  creating new normal, 54–59
  and cultural competence, 138–39
  raising successful and good Black men, 157–58
  and "the talk," 80–83
online support group, 122, 125
oppressive systems, confronting, 109–16
organizations, intersectional considerations for, 185–87

Papa Smurf, son with autism, 29–30, 35, 122, 191
Pappas, son with autism, 30, 32, 52
  class implications of advocacy, 105
  post-diagnosis, 130–31
  raising successful and good Black men, 152–54
  true-to-life experience, 87–92
participants, study, 31–41
partners, helping, 54–59
Paulin, Diana, 120
Pearson, J. N., 103
Peete, Holly Robinson, 80–81
physical therapy (PT), 183
Pianta, R. C., 45–46
pictures of action
  acceptance, 47–51
  community support, 59–61
  creating new normal, 54–59
  religion as coping strategy, 62–64
  self-compassion, 62–64
  strategizing autism learning curve, 51–54
Pierce, N. P., 14
police brutality. *See* brutality, police
Poobie, son with autism, 30, 38–39, 57–58, 81, 100–101, 157, 160–61
Poopy-Doo, son with autism, 29–30, 49, 51, 61, 190
post-diagnosis responses, 43–44, 47–49, 53, 66–68
  acceptance in action, 47–51
  community support, 59–61
  creating new normal, 54–59
  overview of, 45–47
  religion as coping strategy, 62–64
  self-compassion, 64–66
  strategizing autism learning curve, 51–54
post-traumatic slave syndrome, 137
Priest, Michelle, participant, 39, 48–49, 72, 192
  autism in Black churches, 128–29
  building trust with BAMs, 101–2
  coping strategies, 65–66
  creating new normal, 56–57
  on high expectations, 141
  protecting innocence of Black boys, 75–76
  strategizing autism learning curve, 51–53
problem mom. *See* Black autism mothers (BAMs)
providers, intersectional considerations for, 180–83

refrigerator mothers, 10–12
Refrigerator Mothers (documentary), 12
religion, coping, 62–64
representation
  churches, 128–32
  creating cultural spaces, 126–28
  cultural competence, 136–39

representation *(continued)*
  cultural scene, 121–26
  culturally responsive autism care and services, 132–34
  expectations, 139–45
  overview of, 117–21
  sociopolitical consciousness, 135–36
researchers, expectations for, 139–42
Richie, B. E., 90
Rogers, A., 72, 77

sacrifice, special education, 110–12
Sam, son with autism, 30, 39, 48, 53, 65, 76, 101, 102, 121, 192
schools
  after-school care, 2, 142, 144, 161–62
  administrators, 30, 36, 498, 167
  church schools, 130, 178
  environments, 150, 168, 182
  high school, 22, 28, 34–35, 52, 94–95, 112, 114, 128, 154, 160, 190, 192
  homeschool, 149
  middle school, 94, 111–12
  personnel, 95, 100, 104, 108–10, 115
  placements, 3, 12, 64, 94, 95, 105, 182, 190
  relationships, 115
  staff, 59, 96–108, 112, 115, 151, 153, 190
self-compassion, 64–66
service care coordinator, expectations for, 142–45
service disruptions, 143
services, allowance of, 56
Silva, V. T., 12
sociopolitical consciousness, 135–36
Solomon, son with autism, 35, 65, 85, 110, 159
Solomon, O., 13
sons, Black mothers and, 16–18

Sousa, O., 14
special education, involvement with, 97–99
  building trust with BAMs, 99–103
  class implications of advocacy of, 103–6
  giving power back, 114–16
  meetings, 113–14
  sacrifices, 110–12
Sridhar, A., 140
STEAM (science, technology, engineering, arts, and math), 127–28
stereotyping, 141–42
Straiton, D., 140
study
  analysis of data for, 24–25
  data collection methods for, 23–24
  methodology of, 21
  participants in, 21–23. *See also* participants, study
  purpose of, 20–21
superpowers, 41, 152

"the talk," 72, 80–87
teachers, 28, 37, 44, 56, 78, 93, 95–103, 105, 107–8, 112–14, 128, 131, 162, 169, 178, 182–83
"that's not nice," phrase, 156
Thompson, Lisa, participant, 39–40, 57–58, 65, 74, 82–83, 100, 103, 143–44, 151, 155–56, 161–62
threats, 17, 21, 70, 73, 75, 183–84
Tourette's syndrome, 22, 85
true-to-life experience, intersection, 87–92
trust, building, 99–103

Vivanti, Giacomo, 5

warrior mothers, 12–13
Washington Post, 17–18

Washington, H. A., 135
White people, 43, 91
    fragility, 113–14
    warrior mothers, 12–13
Willliams, Kiara, participant, 40–41, 61–62, 99, 108, 152, 155, 192

World War II, 11

Yee, A., 140
Yochim, Chivers, 12

Zimmerman, George, 17

www.ingramcontent.com/pod-product-compliance
Lightning Source LLC
Chambersburg PA
CBHW021942250225
22368CB00011B/90